About the Author

ROZALIND GRAHAM was form
Central YMCA's Training and
she co-developed a postgradua
cise for older adults. She holds a professorship in health science
and applied nutrition and has lectured for several years at
Middlesex University. Rozalind lectures on achieving optimum
health throughout Europe, the United States and in Central
America.

Other titles in *The Daily Telegraph* series

To order further health titles from Robinson,
please see the order form at the back of this book

𝔗𝔥𝔢 𝔇𝔞𝔦𝔩𝔶 𝔗𝔢𝔩𝔢𝔤𝔯𝔞𝔭𝔥

STAY FIT AFTER FIFTY

Your Guide to Well-being in the Second Half of Life

Rozalind Graham

ROBINSON
London

Constable & Robinson Ltd
3 The Lanchesters
162 Fulham Palace Road
London W6 9ER
www.constablerobinson.com

First published in the UK by Robinson,
an imprint of Constable & Robinson Ltd, 2006

A copy of the British Library Cataloguing in Publication
Data is available from the British Library.

ISBN 13: 978-1-84529-144-0
ISBN 10: 1-84529-144-1

Printed and bound in the EU

1 3 5 7 9 10 8 6 4 2

Contents

Introduction

Welcome to a book that is likely to become a treasured and trusted friend. You are about to read something that I hope will leave you feeling informed, inspired and empowered. Whether you are just approaching the second half of your life or are well advanced in years, the opportunity for you to create a greater feeling of well-being awaits you within these pages.

My own search for advice on exercise and healthy living began some 27 years ago. I found that there were generally two types of books available on the subject: those so heavily packed with science that I could hardly lift, much less understand them, and those filled with mostly shallow information based on common sense. It became a life goal for me to educate myself and gain the qualifications and experience necessary not only to reach my own health and fitness goals, but also to help others achieve theirs. I held a vision of creating a book that was solid in its scientific approach without being indigestible, and effective in its practical application.

Over the years, my studies have led me down many interesting and rewarding paths, one of which resulted in me becoming a senior lecturer for London Central YMCA's Training and Development Department. For over a decade, I worked as a Course Director and Assessor of teacher training for fitness professionals throughout the UK. During this time, I co-created – along with fitness expert Susie Dinan – the first postgraduate teacher-training course on exercise for older adults. I also pursued the kind of learning that satisfied my great hunger for knowledge of nutrition and other aspects of healthy living. Eventually these studies culminated in my receiving a professorship in health science and applied nutrition, subjects that I went on to lecture in for several years at London's Middlesex University.

This book is different from the ones I read when I began my training. Its roots are firmly planted in anatomy, physiology and biochemistry. Yet it is filled with practical information that is not to be left on its pages, but is to be applied in your own life. It is a book designed for you personally, to learn from and to use in accordance with your own needs and goals. Most of all, this is a book that will show you how to create a better state of health and fitness for yourself than you are currently experiencing, whatever your health history.

Do you evaluate your own state of health according to the absence or presence of symptoms and signs? If so, I invite you to consider how negative an approach to wellness that is. Health is a glorious state of vibrant exuberance, not just simply the absence of physical discomfort. The term 'dis-ease' can be used to describe times when the body is not 'at ease' due to losing its homeostasis (a word for describing stable internal balance). A loss of homeostasis can be caused when your body is poisoned, disrupted or injured – and/or simply not being provided with its basic requirements for life.

Your state of health is reflected in the vitality of your cells and specific influences affect this. Using your body in ways that it is not designed for – for instance, spending hour after hour sitting at a desk – will result in compromised health. Demanding an intensity of work beyond the ability of any specific aspect of your body is another detrimental influence. Insufficient sleep and rest are a primary cause of devitalized cells. Under-using your physical abilities, however, is also harmful, as can be seen in very sedentary people who may have actually lost significant functional use of their limbs. Indulging in abusive lifestyle habits such as smoking rapidly devitalizes your body on a cellular level, as does living in a polluted environment.

The influence of your psychological attitude upon cellular functioning is increasingly becoming recognized as a key factor in health. Many people become progressively despondent as the years pass, due to our society's negative attitude towards physical maturity. This gradual decline in joy can also contribute to devitalizing our bodies on a cellular level and result in premature physical ageing.

Whatever your age, your body's basic needs must be met in order for it to thrive. Getting older is not a disease, nor is it the cause of disease. The majority of diseases commonly experienced by older adults result from an accumulation of poor dietary and lifestyle habits. It is for this reason that being older and being sick are often seen as synonymous. Heart disease and osteoporosis are excellent examples of conditions that are not the result of simply getting older. Instead, they are the consequence of long-term participation in unhealthy habits. In the absence of excess dietary fats, cardio-respiratory (heart and lung) exertion is actually the aspect of fitness least affected purely by the passing of years. Provided the bloodstream is not over-acidic, bones do not lose their integrity simply because a person is older – their density remains intact right up to the time of death. Our ability to perform activities involving balance, coordination and reaction time is most affected by the natural processes of ageing. Yet even these aspects of fitness can be counteracted by regular participation in sports and recreational activities such as dance, racket sports and yoga.

Young people are typically viewed as fit and healthy simply due to their age, but that assumption is faulty. The youth of today suffer from numerous conditions of ill health as a result of junk food consumption, inactivity and recreational habits such as smoking. Being young does not necessarily mean you are fit, just as being old does not necessarily mean you are unfit. Many active older adults are far fitter than some inactive youngsters are. Most aspects of physical decline that we experience as we get older are due to nothing more than inactivity and poor diet. The ageing process does not bring them about.

One of the most talked about changes that take place as we age is hormone activity. Just as the adolescent experiences hormonal shifts, the older adult body also undergoes changes within the endocrine (hormone) system. In neither case is this natural occurrence a manifestation of disease, but rather the natural evolution of the human organism as it experiences the passage of time. It is further amiss to believe that hormonal changes are exclusive to women – they are not. As both men and women grow older, the glands of the endocrine system produce less of certain hormones. In healthy individuals, such changes produce few or no symptoms. For a person who is already in a poor state of health prior to these changes, however, the symptoms can be distressing and uncomfortable.

Levels of testosterone and aldosterone drop naturally in men as they get older. A reduction in testosterone may result in a loss of muscle mass, but the effect this has on an individual depends on how strong they were in the first place. An older man whose work regularly demands heavy manual labour, or who performs callisthenics or participates in weight training, will have far greater muscular bulk than a sedentary youngster will.

Reduced testosterone also contributes to a drop in the metabolic rate (the speed at which biochemical reactions occur within the body). This can lead to a gain in body fat in men who lead sedentary lifestyles. By developing regular exercise and healthy eating habits, a man can counteract the slowing of metabolism and maintain a healthy body composition.

Reductions in the rate at which nutrients are converted to fuel within the muscles of older men and women used to be considered age-related. However, studies now reveal that this is not the case. It has been concluded that this reduced efficiency results from inactivity rather than from the passage of time.

A working knowledge of natural bodily changes can help us approach things in better ways. For example, the drop in aldosterone that naturally occurs in older men results in their being less able to cool themselves down by sweating, because this hormone is responsible for promoting the retention of sodium, potassium and water by the kidneys. Heatstroke is therefore more liable to occur. Older men need to allow for this by taking extra care to keep well hydrated, especially when exerting themselves in hot weather.

For women, it is primarily progesterone production that diminishes with age. As this hormone keeps oestrogen in check, it is vital not to allow excess oestrogen to become a problem. Too much circulating oestrogen can cause many serious conditions including cancer of the breast, cervix and uterus. Ways to combat this include avoiding exposure to the oestrogen mimics known as xenoestrogens, which are found in some foods and many household products, and maintaining a healthy body weight via correct diet and regular exercise. On the other hand, fruits and vegetables are abundant in substances known as phytoestrogens. These substances have the remarkable capacity to block excess oestrogens (including xenoestrogens) from the receptor sites, while also being so similar to human oestrogens that they can be used by the body in the event of an oestrogen deficiency.

Over the years, scientists have collected much evidence indicating that regular exercise increases both longevity and quality of life. One of the most definitive studies in this respect was conducted at Harvard and involved 16,936 graduates aged 35 to 74. The researchers used a questionnaire to ascertain the general health and lifestyle habits of each person in the study. Exercise was recorded as calories expended. Those who expended 2,000 calories per week exercising had mortality rates 25 to 30 per cent lower than those who were less physically active. This amount of calorie expenditure translates into only one hour of brisk walking per day.

One of the greatest obstacles to an older person's participation in exercise can be society's attitudes and expectations toward ageing. The view is usually taken that older adults are structurally fragile, and the older they become the more sedentary their lifestyle should be. One ageing athlete was heard to say that the only reason he cut back on his training was that he believed he was too decrepit to achieve the athleticism he was demonstrating. Yet many so-called miracles have been shown in all corners of the globe. Jean Borotra and Kitty Godfry were top-rated tennis players who were still playing when they were in their nineties. Edward Western was a man who walked across the USA and back in his mid-seventies. At the age of 60, a man named Ron Taylor ran 100m in 11.3 seconds. And Cliff Young, who was 61 years young at the time, won the first Sydney to Melbourne race.

You may be thinking that there are always exceptions, but in nature a rule is a rule. If the passing of years, by natural law, resulted in our becoming decrepit by the sixth decade, then none of the above achievements could have occurred.

Ask a ten-year-old child if she or he is looking forward to being over 40 and it's unlikely the response will be positive. In our culture, the mature years are portrayed as a time of degeneration of body and mind. Yet it does not have to be that way. With the right education, guidance and resources you can create a magnificently different experience for yourself. By adopting a genuinely healthful lifestyle, including the safe and effective exercise habits described in this book, you can transform the years ahead into a time of supreme personal excellence.

Older age should be a time of celebration, as the latter years of life carry with them the promise of greater wisdom, courage and joy.

The autumn of our fifth decade has its own unique beauty equal to that of any springtime, and the winter of our truly older age can be nothing short of magical. The secret of graceful and joyous ageing is to seek out knowledge of how best to look after yourself and then to apply that information with a youthful mentality. In doing so, you will free yourself from the negative expectations of older age and go on to fulfill your potential while enjoying your remarkable life to the fullest.

Chapter One outlines what your body needs in order to be healthy and presents you with a picture of what constitutes healthful living. This is followed by advice on how to make the necessary changes in your lifestyle so that you can create your own health. The chapter concludes with a quiz, enabling you to evaluate your current lifestyle choices. (You can use this quiz repeatedly in the future to measure your progress.)

In Chapter Two, we take an in-depth look at the natural bodily changes that occur as we age, plus the implications that these changes have for our health, well-being and fitness potential.

Chapter Three introduces the five components of fitness and provides an inspiring look at the positive and powerful difference regular exercise can make to the maturing body.

Chapter Four takes you through the steps necessary to launch into a new exercise program. A quiz is included to enable you to evaluate your current level of fitness and select an appropriate starting intensity and duration. In this chapter you will also find guidance on goal-setting and planning your own progressive fitness program.

Once you have studied Chapter Four and identified your fitness level, you are ready to begin the exercises set out in Chapter Five. These are grouped according to intensity and difficulty, and correlate with your score on the fitness quiz. In providing you with a comprehensive program of basic key exercises suitable for your current fitness level, these exercises will give you a good start and may become long-term favourites for you to return to whenever you choose.

For those of you with special health concerns, I encourage you to read Chapter Six before beginning any new exercise regime. In this chapter, you will find information about specific health conditions that are most common to older bodies. You will learn about exercises that can help support healing, as well as the kinds of exercise to avoid so as not to exacerbate any existing conditions.

Chapter Seven introduces you to sports and recreational activities that provide exercise opportunities. Recommendations are given on how to get the most physical benefit out of your participation, along with advice on specific approaches to warming up beforehand and cooling down afterwards.

At the end of the book, there is a section explaining the exercise implications of the most commonly prescribed medications. If you are currently taking any drugs, I recommend that you turn to this section so that you can become familiar with how they may affect your ability to undertake an exercise program /or the outcome of your training. If you are in any doubt, please consult your heath-care professional. At the back of the book you will also find a list of useful organizations and other resources.

I do not claim that this book is definitive, or that it is the only health and fitness book you will need. Scientific facts are being discovered all the time, along with new questions that challenge long-held beliefs. To present this work as anything other than an honest contribution to the subject would be to declare myself as a student who is no longer learning. It is said that it is only when we stop learning that we become old. I invite you to read on and learn how you can achieve a vibrant state of health and well being throughout the second half of your life.

Chapter 1
Creating a Healthy Lifestyle

The recipe for health has a very specific list of ingredients, all of which must be present in the proper proportions if health is to be your outcome. An excess of one ingredient cannot make up for the absence or insufficiency of another, nor can any drug, potion, supplement, elixir or other modality negate an unhealthful diet or lifestyle. Starting an exercise programme without paying proper attention to the other essential elements of a healthy living will be self-defeating in the long term. This chapter introduces you to the key components of health creation and explains how exercise plays an integral role in boosting your overall vitality and sense of well-being.

If you have even a mild interest in gardening, then you are probably aware that plants have specific needs that must be met if they are to flourish. The location, environment, soil type, exposure to sunlight, water, nutrients, and many other aspects of their care must be taken into consideration if the gardener is to be successful. If any one of these needs is not met – or if the plant is subjected to poisons or damage – it will sicken and die. Similarly, your body has its own unique needs that must be met if it is to thrive. Anything that poisons, damages or harms your body in any way should be actively avoided if health is your goal.

Your basic needs for health include:

- Pure air to breathe
- Pure water to drink
- Sufficient sleep
- The correct type, quantity and quality of foods
- Sufficient exercise
- Appropriate exposure to full-spectrum sunlight
- A positive mental outlook and emotionally healthy relationships.

Living in the Western world we face a wide range of health challenges. Some you can avoid, such as tobacco and alcohol; some you cannot, such as smog. You need to make the healthiest choices for yourself within the limitations of your chosen living location.

Breathing Free

The importance of breathing fresh, unpolluted air is probably the most underestimated aspect of personal health care. Researchers working for *National Geographic* magazine conducted a study of peoples of the world with the longest life expectancies. Apart from the fact that all the groups studied eat a largely, or exclusively, vegetarian diet, the one thing they all have in common is that they live at a high altitude where the air is exceptionally clean.

The Sources of Air Pollution

The Global Environment Monitoring System (GEMS), set up by the United Nations and working in conjunction with the World Health Organization, estimates that 1.2 billion inhabitants of cities across the globe are exposed to air pollutants at levels sufficient to damage their health. Most major air pollutants result from the burning of fossil fuels, a large proportion of which are produced by car emissions and domestic cooking stoves.

Consider ways in which you can reduce your own impact on air pollution – can you use the car less for example, and take the opportunity to reap some exercise benefit at the same time by walking or cycling instead?

We can also subject ourselves to a range of pollutants in our own homes. The overuse of powerful chemical cleaning products, for instance, can create a cocktail effect that can poison the body and cause the bronchiole tubes to become irritated and inflamed. Try to minimize the use of chemicals and, if you do use them, air the room well during and after use.

Despite these airborne assaults to our systems, amongst the many benefits of regular aerobic exercise is that it improves our ability to eliminate toxins including carbon dioxide from our systems. Carbon dioxide is constantly manufactured by your body as a by-product of your metabolic processes and is eliminated from your system every time you exhale. Aerobic exercise improves the functioning and efficiency of your entire respiratory system.

As you grow older, there is a tendency for you to breathe less deeply, which is primarily due to a reduction in the elasticity of your respiratory system. As a result, you will gradually have an increased residual volume (the amounts of air left in your lungs after each exhale). A higher residual volume renders you more vulnerable to being poisoned by airborne toxins. By keeping yourself aerobically fit, you can reduce your residual volume and so better protect yourself from air pollution. This is yet another reason why it makes good sense to exercise!

Ways to Protect Yourself from Air Pollutants

1. Do not inhale tobacco, either directly or passively.
2. Stand upwind if pumping fuel into your vehicle.
3. Minimize time spent driving, especially in heavy traffic.
4. Minimize the use of a tumble-dryer. Dry clothes in the sun whenever possible, or get a drip-dry clothes dryer that fits over your bath.
5. Ensure adequate ventilation in enclosed spaces, especially when sharing that space with a group of other people.
6. Sleep with a window open.
7. If you eat cooked food, ensure your kitchen is especially well ventilated while you are cooking
8. Improve the general ventilation of your home and workplace.
9. Keep gas appliances in good repair.
10. Distinguish which household cleaning products you really need from those that manufacturers insist you need. Replace ones you need with those manufactured by companies whose selling point is their product's environmental friendliness (resources are listed at the back of the book), or revert to your great-grandmother's homemade recipes for cleaning products, such as vinegar to clean windows.
11. Reconsider your use of mothballs, which contain highly toxic chemicals such as paradichlorobenzene. Sachets of any of the following are excellent alternatives: dried lavender, equal parts of rosemary and mint, whole peppercorns or wood chips soaked in cedar oil.

12. The rate of mucus production within your nose is just enough to keep the passageways moist. If your nose is healthy, it replaces its mucus secretions every 20 minutes. If you spend time in an overheated home or office, your nasal mucus will dry out and you will be less resistant to diseases of the respiratory tract. When the temperature of your environment makes it necessary to add artificial heat, it is a wise idea simultaneously to increase the humidity. There are various ways that you can do this, but the simplest is to place a large container of water in the room. Aim to maintain indoor humidity levels of between 30 and 50 per cent.

13. Make the necessary changes in your diet (such as minimizing the amount of dairy products you eat) to eliminate congestive mucus so that you can breathe freely through your nose. The nasal passageways play an important part in the filtering, warming and humidifying of incoming air.

14. Buy paints from a manufacturer whose selling point is their product's low toxicity (see Appendix 2) and keep paint stripper tightly sealed and well away from enclosed living areas.

15. Freshen the air by getting rid of air fresheners. Many of these products contain highly toxic chemicals such as naphthalene, phenol, cresol, ethanol, xylene and formaldehyde. If there is a foul smell in the air, open a window. Empty household waste receptacles and dustbins frequently and keep them clean. Sprinkling half a cup of borax in the bottom of your dustbin will inhibit the growth of odour-producing moulds and bacteria. Fragrant herbs and flowers are a delightful addition to any home or office. Consider placing sachets or little dishes of dried herbs, rose petals or lavender where unpleasant odours are a problem.

Sleeping Your Way to Health and Vitality

It has been estimated that your brain's workload is comparable to a telephone operator co-ordinating calls from 36,000 planets, each with a population of four billion. Knowing that your brain is this intelligent could improve your self-esteem and personal pride no end!

Every second of your life your body's cells send millions of messages to your brain, informing it of their condition. This constant relay of information enables your brain to monitor all bodily processes and send appropriate demands back to the cells in order to maintain homeostasis (a constant state of internal balance). Data is received, processed and responded to at a speed and efficiency far beyond the capacity of any computer.

Being physically active, adapting to environmental changes, cleaning out toxic wastes, conducting emotions, healing damaged tissues and managing normal metabolic functions and physiological processes are just a few examples of how your nervous energy gets used up.

What Happens as You Sleep

During sleep, you recharge your nervous energy and accelerate the healing and repair of any damaged tissues. The processes of detoxification and elimination also intensify as you sleep and psychological data that you have accumulated throughout the day is processed. If you sleep in a stressful or fretful way, you will not reach the deeper levels of sleep, resulting in a poor quality – and ineffective – night's rest.

The Dangers of Being Under-slept

When under-slept, the body's central nervous system is undercharged, resulting in the brain being compromised in its ability to co-ordinate the workings of the body, including all aspects of immune functioning.

Sleep and Dietary Habits

Being under-slept is a major cause of unhealthful eating habits. If you feel tired throughout the day, you are far more liable to overeat in an attempt to increase your energy, but this will always be counter-productive. Although the act of eating may result in temporary immediate stimulation, the task of digesting food requires your body to expend energy. The aftermath of a heavy meal will always be an even deeper state of tiredness. Being tired can lead you to crave foods containing refined sugar. Due to the rapidity with which these sugars enter your bloodstream, the consumption of them will cause a hyperactive state for a very short period of time. This will always be followed by a plummeting in your energy levels. The same applies if you take other stimulants such as coffee, tea or chocolate. Tiredness may cause you to rely on fast foods, junk foods or convenience foods rather than preparing healthy meals. The long-term consequences of such choices include a progressive deepening of your body's exhaustion. The good news is that here, too, exercise can help. Exercise can release psychologically induced muscular tension, and help you to relax your mind – both vital ingredients for helping you get a good night's sleep.

Ten Guidelines for Rejuvenating Sleep

1. Learn how to better manage your stress so that you can fully relax when you go to bed at night.
2. Do your exercise about five hours before you intend to sleep. The drop in body temperature that typically occurs approximately this long after vigorous exercise helps to induce sleep.
3. Develop night-time rituals or a routine of preparation for bed. This can help you to mentally switch off from the day and prepare you for superior quality sleep.
4. Eat healthily and avoid stimulants such as caffeine and sugary foods.
5. Avoid emotional stimulation immediately prior to sleep. Participate only in peaceful recreational activities during the evening and postpone all challenging interactions for another day.
6. Once in bed, the practice of deliberately and methodically relaxing your muscles is very effective in securing quality sleep. A good yoga teacher or stress management coach can help you learn how to do this.
7. Ensure that your sleeping environment is dark, quiet, ventilated and comfortable.
8. If you have difficulty getting to sleep, do not 'try' to sleep but focus instead on simply relaxing.
9. If you still can't sleep, get up from your bed and read or listen to music until you are more relaxed so as not to associate the bed with restlessness and distress.
10. If a racing mind prevents you from sleeping, allow yourself to think of anything; providing it is nothing to do with the past, and nothing to do with the future. This is a very effective way of dissolving stress by being present moment to moment.

Light Up Your Life

Sunlight is as necessary to your health as air and water. Your body is affected by full-spectrum sunlight in far more ways than you might realize. Insufficient exposure to it will disrupt your physiological functioning. Your libido, appetite, emotional health, cellular normality – as well as your ability to utilize nutrients from the foods that you eat – are all affected by sunlight.

The rays of the sun are needed to keep your bones strong. This is because calcium is a major constituent of bone and your body cannot process calcium without the presence of sufficient vitamin D. Sunlight enables your body to synthesize vitamin D, which is why it is referred to as the 'sunshine vitamin'.

Vitamin D is also needed for the absorption of phosphorous, an important mineral that your body uses for many things including the assimilation of niacin (vitamin B3). Niacin is essential for orgasmic sexual experience. When your exposure to sunlight is insufficient, the consequent reduction in phosphorous absorption can result in your experiencing severely diminished, or absent, libido.

A lack of natural light disrupts the functioning of your hypothalamus, a small region of your brain situated between its two hemispheres. The hypothalamus enables communications between your central and autonomic nervous systems to take place. It also connects your nervous system to your hormone-producing glands and plays a major role in the switching on and off of your appetite. During times of sunlight deprivation, you may experience disrupted eating habits that either manifest as overeating or a diminished desire for food. Due to the influence of sunlight on your body's production of melatonin (a hormone) and serotonin (a neurotransmitter), your mood will be adversely affected by a lack of full-spectrum sunlight entering your eyes. This is one of the reasons why wearing sunglasses is not recommended, except when you need to protect your eyes from the glare of reflected sun (such as when skiing) or to shade your vision for safe driving.

Your body's ability to protect itself is yet another aspect of health that is dependent on sunlight. Full-spectrum sunlight enables your body to increase the production and activity of its defences. The health of your immune system is boosted by exposure to sunlight.

Anything that is good for you is only good in appropriate amounts. The 'more is better' motto, within any aspect of health care, is unhealthful. Exposure to sun is no exception to this rule. It is important to avoid burning the skin and fair-skinned people need to be particularly careful about over-exposure. If you are in the tropics, stay out of the sun between 10am and 4pm, or cover up with breathable clothing and a hat.

Happy Thoughts

An upward spiral to a healthy and happy future depends as much upon nurturing your thoughts as it does on nurturing your physical body. The way you process your world, all your perceptions and interpretations of events, contribute to creating your emotions. In turn, your emotional state has a powerful influence on your physical health.

According to Kenneth Pelletier, a senior clinical fellow at the Centre for Disease Prevention at Stanford University Medical School:

> Emotional states ranging from love and compassion to fear and anger can trigger chain reactions that affect blood chemistry, heart rate, and the activity of every cell and organ system in the body – from the stomach and gastrointestinal tract to the immune system. All of that is now indisputable fact.

A famous study conducted by Harvard psychologist Walter B. Cannon revealed the consistent ways in which the body reacts, on a physical level, to perceived stressors. Cannon named this collection of physical changes the Fight or Flight Response. His studies involved looking at catecholamines, a collection of hormones secreted by the body when under stress. Epinephrine (also known as adrenaline) is the best known of the catecholamines. It is produced by the adrenal glands, situated on the top of each kidney. Individuals suffering from chronic stress are often referred to as suffering from adrenal exhaustion.

Until recently, the medical profession considered the central nervous system and immune functioning to be independent and separate entities. There is, however, substantial evidence to show that they are directly related. Nerve endings have been found in the thymus, lymph nodes, spleen and bone marrow, structures that play fundamental roles in immunity. It seems that the immune cells respond directly to chemicals once thought to affect only the nervous system. It has also become apparent that nerve cells respond to chemical messengers secreted by the immune system.

Heartfelt Emotions

Back in 1936, it was discovered that the proliferation of certain immune cells, known as eosinophilia, was associated with heart failure. The fact that these cells are influenced by psychological factors has led to an entirely new area of research. Scientists are now examining the links between emotions and the physiological functioning of the heart. Studies have revealed that changes triggered by negative emotional states can affect the heart in the following ways.

- *Raising blood pressure* Various stressors, ranging from mental arithmetic to physical discomfort, have been shown to induce elevated blood pressure in both healthy individuals and people with borderline high blood pressure. Increases are greater, and more prolonged, for those individuals with borderline or pre-existing hypertension.
- *Spasms of the coronary arteries* Mental stress, such as doing complex math (a standard experimental stressor), have been shown to induce a spasm, or sudden constriction, of the coronary arteries.
- *Changes in the blood* Stress hormones may indirectly increase the blood's tendency to clot and raise the blood cholesterol level.

All this provides a powerful argument for the importance of attending to your emotional happiness – whether this be through stress reduction, making more opportunities for pursuing interests and pastimes that truly stimulate and fulfil you, or simply finding better ways to relax. Regular exercise can help in all three areas.

The years of your life bring you endless opportunities to grow in wisdom and inner peace. Some of those opportunities can be a challenge to experience; others can be a joy. The fast pace of westernized life, with its noise and distractions, can be the enemy of your serenity. Taking time in solitude and quiet can be your soul's healer and the doctor of your disquiet. Just a few moments each day, spent in silence, or the company of the gentle sounds of nature, can nourish your spirit like a cool glass of water on a hot day. Becoming healthy and fit involves tapping into the limit-less love that lies within you, for it is within this love that true peace awaits you.

Living Clean, Living Well

Many factors influence how quickly your body ages and degener-ates. The extent that you are exposed to environmental toxins is a major consideration, and one of your most direct contacts with such things are the toiletries and cosmetics that you use. All of these items are toxic to some degree. There are probably more products in your bathroom that you absolutely do not need than in any other room in your home.

It is possible for you to take some of the most commonly used items and set about transforming your bathroom from a chem-istry lab into a health sanctuary! The table below summarizes the chemicals found in them and suggests natural alternatives.

Product	Possible ingredients	Alternatives
Anti-dandruff shampoo	Selenium sulphide and resorcinol	Natural liquid soap to wash hair and diluted lemon juice to rinse.
Deodorant and anti-perspirant	Aluminium chlorohydrate, triclosan	Wash regularly, and wear natural, breathable fibres. Add a few drops of essential oil such as sage, rosemary or cinnamon to distilled water and spray your underarms.
Toothpaste	Formaldehyde, saccharine, polyvinylpyrrolid plastics	Rinse mouth with plain water after each meal. Floss regularly. Mix 1 teaspoon of water with 1 teaspoon of essential oil of peppermint or clove as a toothpaste alternative.

Hair colourant	Chemicals known as xenoestrogens	Henna for dark hair, or cooled camomile tea mixed with the juice of 1 lemon or lime for light hair.
Hairspray and styling mousse	Formaldehyde, polyvinylpyrrolidone plastic	Cut two unpeeled oranges into slices, and then boil them in four cups of water until half the water has evaporated. Pour the liquid through a sieve, discarding the orange flesh and peel. Add a teaspoon of lemon juice to the orange water and then pour it into a spray bottle.
Perfumes and aftershaves	Formaldehyde, phenol, trichloroethylene, and creosol	Use essential oils. Sandalwood is the preferred scent of many health-seeking men. Many women prefer the beautiful scent of pure rose or jasmine. Most essential oils need to be mixed with a little carrier oil, such as jojoba, almond or grape seed, before being applied to the skin.
Talcum powder	Possible contamination with silica, asbestos	Plain rice starch combined with dried and ground lavender.

Becoming a Smoke-free Zone

The lethal effects of tobacco use have been known for decades. Back in March 1938, an article entitled 'Tobacco Smoking and Longevity' by Dr Raymond Pearl of John Hopkins University stated, 'Statistics show that a heavy smoker loses from his or her lifespan 34.6 minutes for each cigarette he smokes.'

You may consider yourself a non-smoker, but every time you can smell someone else's tobacco smoke, you also are inhaling it. In 1988, the Independent Scientific Committee on Smoking and

Health, an advisory body to the government, examined all the scientific data available on the effects of passive smoking and concluded that side-stream inhalation did significantly increase the risk of lung cancer. The committee estimated that passive smoking might be responsible for hundreds of lung cancer deaths per year in the UK.

There is an iron-rich compound circulating in your blood called haemoglobin. As you inhale, oxygen reaches the alveoli of your lungs, where it passes into the blood and attaches to the haemoglobin in order to be transported around your body. Tobacco smoke contains the deadly toxic gas carbon monoxide, which is highly attracted to haemoglobin. When carbon monoxide is inhaled, it passes into the blood from the alveoli and effectively hijacks the haemoglobin. All smokers are oxygen starved in this way; about 20 per cent of their red blood cells are saturated with carbon monoxide instead of oxygen.

Once in your circulation, carbon monoxide gains access to every cell in your body and poisons them. Carbon monoxide also severely damages your arteries. It is so caustic that the linings of your blood vessels become inflamed by its presence in the circulating blood. Once inflamed, your vessel walls are predisposed to the adherence of fatty deposits and cholesterol that accumulate to impede, and eventually block, your blood flow. This can result in a heart attack or stroke.

Another highly poisonous substance contained in tobacco smoke is nicotine. Nicotine causes the arteries to constrict, further reducing the oxygen supply to the entire body, including the heart and brain. Nicotine also causes the blood to become sticky, which can lead to death through the formation of blood clots.

A wide range of respiratory diseases result from smoking, including chronic bronchitis and lung cancer. Smoking directly causes almost all cases of emphysema.

Smoking and Cancer

Tobacco inhalation is known to contribute to causing all types of cancer, especially of the lungs. According to the Health Education Authority, smoking directly causes nine out of every ten deaths from lung cancer. In England alone, this amounts to a staggering 29,000 deaths per year. It has been estimated that you only need to smoke one cigarette per day to increase the likelihood of dying from lung cancer by 800 per cent. Cancer of the tongue and pharynx are also caused almost exclusively by smoking. In addition, smoking reduces the effectiveness of your immune system, compromises the effectiveness of your digestive system and can contribute to osteoporosis and other bone diseases.

The Good News about Not Smoking!

As soon as you begin to get smoke out of your life, your body will set about cleansing itself of tobacco's noxious poisons. The speed and degree to which it can accomplish this depends on many factors, including the number of years you have been smoking and how much you smoked each day. By eating a healthy diet, getting ample sleep and exercising regularly, you will enhance your recovery. Farewell to smoking also means farewell to:

- Foul-smelling breath, hair and clothing
- Stained teeth and fingers
- Phlegm and smokers cough
- Wrinkled skin and premature ageing.

Hello to pure air also means hello to:

- An improved sense of taste and smell
- Easier breathing on exertion
- A vast improvement in health status
- More money.

If you are a smoker, getting rid of your smoking habit is the single most important thing you can do for your health.

Alcohol in Focus

For optimum health it is also very important to look at reducing your alcohol intake. Alcohol is a powerful drug and is treated as toxic by your body. The short-term effects of heavy drinking include an upset stomach, diarrhoea, anaemia and dry skin. Long-term effects include many serious conditions including liver damage, problems with attention, thinking and memory.

The British Medical Association (BMA) reports that liver disorders (such as fatty liver), hepatitis (where individual liver cells are destroyed and there is inflammation and scarring of the liver) and cirrhosis are far more common amongst heavy drinkers. They also document that heavy drinkers suffer from higher-than-average rates of gastritis, pancreatitis (inflammation of the pancreas), peptic ulcers and cancers of the mouth, tongue, pharynx, larynx, oesophagus and stomach.

Having a 'fatty liver' is reversible, but once the condition has gone on to become cirrhosis, it is not. According to the BMA, a daily average intake of 45ml of alcohol (four single whiskies or four glasses of wine) puts you at a high risk of this disease.[1]

Alcohol and Osteoporosis

It is important to be aware that alcohol consumption is a major contributory cause of osteoporosis. This is because:

1. It impairs your liver's ability to activate vitamin D, without which you cannot absorb calcium.
2. The acidifying effect alcohol has on your blood results in the alkaline mineral calcium being leached from your bones in order to return the blood pH to normal.

Alcohol and Your Athletic Performance

If you drink alcohol, it will affect your ability to exercise in the following ways:

1. Reduce your coordination, reaction time, balance and judgement of distance, space and time.
2. Reduce your strength, power, speed and endurance.
3. Reduce your ability to regulate your body temperature.
4. Reduce your blood sugar levels and increase your risk of hypoglycaemia.
5. Increase your excretion of water, resulting in dehydration.
6. Increase your risk of accident and injury.

The degree to which alcohol damages your health will always be equal to the quantity consumed. Remembering this will prevent you from ever feeling disappointed with the results of your choices.

Healthy Eating

This is such an important topic it could profitably have its own chapter. So much strong scientific evidence is now emerging about the link between diet and disease that it really is essential to become well informed. Unfortunately it is beyond the scope of this book to describe in detail all the health benefits of sensible eating, but the list of resources in Appendix 2 will guide you to some excellent websites and books.

Fruit and Vegetables as the Basis of Your Diet

Scientific research and the evidence of disease patterns around the world show very clearly that the healthiest diets are those high in fruit and vegetables and lower in total fat. The 1997 report *Food, Nutrition and the Prevention of Cancer* published by the World Cancer Research Fund in association with the American Institute for Cancer Research, concluded that 'Evidence of dietary protection against cancer is strongest and most consistent for diets high in vegetables and fruits.'

It is not just cancer that can be prevented by dietary change – the incidence of heart disease, type 2 diabetes and osteoporosis are all much lower in the rural population of countries such as China and Japan, where diet is still based on traditional plant foods. We can make these changes in our daily diets and reap similar benefits. One study conducted by researchers in Australia revealed that when people adopted a vegetarian diet for six weeks, there was a significant drop in their blood pressure. After returning to a diet that included meat and dairy foods, their blood pressure went back up.[2] On average, the systolic blood pressure of vegetarians is eight to nine points lower, and the diastolic six to eight points lower, than amongst people eating a standard western diet.[3]

A properly designed diet of raw fresh fruits and vegetables provides the perfect nutritional match for the needs of the human body. These foods provide carbohydrates, fats, proteins, vitamins, minerals, fibre and water all in appropriate ratios.

The Importance of Wholefoods

Refined foods are those that have had most of their fibre, or other nutrients, removed; white bread and fruit juices are two such examples. The opposite of a refined food is one that is whole, with its full nutrient package still intact.

Fibre is found only in plant foods – no meat or dairy products contain any fibre. Also known as 'bulk' or 'roughage', it is an essential nutrient for health. One role of fibre is to promote peristalsis, the waves of muscular contraction that usher food through your intestinal tract. If you habitually consume a diet that is low in fibre, your intestinal musculature will atrophy. This results in food passing too slowly through your intestines, leading to problems ranging from constipation and malabsorption of food to colon cancer.

Pectin and gum are specific types of fibres present in fruits and vegetables that are especially important for your health. These water-soluble fibres help to reduce cholesterol levels by binding with it, along with bile salts, with the result that all three substances leave the body together. This has a two-fold benefit: not only will you excrete unwanted cholesterol, but your body will also use up more cholesterol in remaking the lost bile salts. The result is a further reduction in your circulating level of cholesterol. Another role of fibre is to moderate the release of monosaccharides (simple sugars) into your bloodstream. A lack of fibre can result in sharp rises and falls in your blood sugar level, causing you to experience mood swings, lethargy and even hypoglycaemia and diabetes. Fibre also absorbs water while in the stomach, leaving you to feeling full sooner and reducing the possibility of you overeating.

It is important to eat fruit and vegetables raw, as far as possible, to preserve the nutrients within them. Choosing organic foods is important in order to minimize your exposure to pesticides and toxic chemical fertilizers.

The other important issue for healthy eating is the reduction of salt in your diet. Research has shown that high blood pressure and a higher risk of stomach cancer are both associated with high salt intake. Try to minimize your intake of processed foods, which often have a high salt content and concentrate on natural, whole foods.

The Dangers of Excess Fat

Excess fat in the diet causes more suffering and premature deaths than any other single dietary influence upon human health. Much of the fat consumed by westernized populations comes from meat and dairy sources, but even plant fats, if eaten in excess, can cause devastating results. All well-educated nutritional and dietary experts are in agreement that your body only requires between 7 and 10 per cent of your total calorie intake in a day to come from fats. The average fat consumption amongst Europeans and Americans is over 40 per cent. Excess dietary fat is a key contributor to three of the leading causes of premature death in our society – cancer, heart disease and diabetes. If you are only ready to make one change in your dietary habits, I encourage you to reduce your overall intake of fats. The easiest and simplest way to do this is to increase your consumption of fruits and vegetables. These foods typically contain between one 1 and 10 per cent of their calories as fat, compared to the 45 to 95 per cent present in most meat and dairy meals.

The Dangers of Excess Food

It's interesting to note that the longest-lived peoples of the world have body weights that would be considered underweight according to Western standards. Being overweight impacts upon more than just your appearance. Being obese increases your risk of high blood pressure, stroke and diabetes. Excess weight in men is associated with an increased risk of cancer of the rectum, colon, and prostate. Amongst women, excess weight gain increases the risk of breast, uterine, and cervical cancer. The road to obesity is also the road to premature ageing, gallstones, heart disease, arthritis and digestive disorders. In short, being obese increases your risk of becoming seriously ill.

Your body is composed of different types of tissue. Lean tissue is a term used to collectively describe those tissues other than fat such as muscle and bone. Adipose tissue is the correct term for stores of body fat. Your total body weight (TBW) is the sum total weight of your entire body. There are various methods of ascertaining what percentage of your TBW is made up of fat tissue. Each method has its advantages and disadvantages. The use of bioimpedance scales, similar to ordinary bathroom scales, give you your body fat percentage as well as your total body weight. They are probably the most accurate in relation to practical convenience.

Ideal ranges for body fat are between 4 and 10 per cent for men and between 12 and 18 per cent for women. Most authorities state them as being higher than this, with recommendations for men being up to 20 per cent and women up to 25 per cent. This is due to the fact that the average person in Western society so far exceeds the ideal that a compromise is offered.

Excess body fat predisposes a person to a multitude of serious degenerative conditions. Just because a person weighs lighter on the scale, it is no guarantee that they have a healthy muscle-to-fat ratio. Insufficient muscle mass leads to a sluggish metabolism, compromised lymphatic functioning, skeletal instability, and poor posture. The state of being under-muscled is as common a problem as being over-fat. A healthy body is lean and strong.

Whenever the TBW exceeds that for which a person's skeletal frame was designed to carry, undue strain is placed upon the weight-bearing joints, including the lower spine. This can result in degeneration of the joints, and conditions such as osteoarthritis.

The number of calories you require in order to maintain your weight is directly related to the amount you exercise. Generally, if your body is using a greater number of calories than are being taken in, weight loss will occur. If calories are consumed beyond that needed by the body's activities, an increase in weight will be the result.

There are many reasons why some people habitually overeat. In most cases, greed has very little, if anything, to do with it. The most common reason people consume food in excess is because it can effectively be used to numb emotional pain. Another common, but mostly unrecognized cause is malnutrition. When the diet is deficient in available nutrients, the body will continue to initiate hunger in an attempt to have its needs met. Even in cases where the diet is sufficient, a poor ability to digest or assimilate food can result in malnutrition and the triggering of an ever-present hunger.

Other reasons for over-eating include consuming food in an attempt to overcome fatigue, eating to resolve boredom, eating to satisfy addictive cravings, and eating as a replacement for smoking. Interestingly, a lack of exercise can also result in overeating. This is due to the fact that lethargy breeds fatigue, and fatigue seeks stimulation. So introducing exercise into your life will not only burn up excess calories — it can also address the reasons why you may be overeating.

Creating Health

So how do you shape up in terms of the various components of health? Try the following quiz for a quick guide.

How Healthy is <u>Your</u> Lifestyle?

1) Do you smoke any form of tobacco?
   a) Yes, daily
   b) Not daily, but few weeks are smoke-free
   c) Rarely – some months are smoke free
   d) No, never

2) How many of the following are *totally* tobacco smoke-free zones? Your living environment; your working environment; your social environment; your travelling environments.
   a) Only one
   b) Two
   c) Three
   d) All four

3) How much time do you spend, on average, travelling in heavy traffic in a vehicle on the road?
   a) Over 1 hour per day
   b) Over 30 minutes per day
   c) Less than 30 minutes per day
   d) Less than 30 minutes per month

4) On average, how many hours of actual sleep do you get within every 24-hour period?
   a) Less than 6 hours
   b) 6–7 hours

    c) 7–8 hours

    d) 8 hours or more

5) Do you wake up naturally, or by some other means?

    a) An alarm, another person, or a pet usually awakens me

    b) I set an alarm, but wake up before it goes off

    c) I usually awaken naturally and only arrange to be awakened by an alarm or another person on occasions when it is necessary

    d) I always wake up naturally

6) How much time do you spend outside in the sun with a significant amount of your skin exposed to its natural light?

    a) At all times, I avoid exposing myself to the sun

    b) A couple of weeks per year on holiday and weekends when it is sunny

    c) At least an hour a day for at least six months of the year

    d) At least an hour most days of the year

7) How would you rate your overall levels of stress?

    a) I feel stressed and anxious all the time – I'm a nervous wreck

    b) I often feel worried about things and don't always sleep well

    c) Occasionally I'm a little stressed and anxious, but I feel it's under control

    d) Generally speaking I'm calm and happy

8) How often do you drink alcohol?

    a) Over three units on a daily basis

    b) A couple of units three or four times a week

    c) Maybe once a week or just on special occasions

    d) I never drink alcohol

9) My relationships are:
   a) Unhappy and stressful
   b) On the whole okay
   c) Generally happy
   d) Truly rewarding and fulfilling

10) On average, how many of your meals each day include meat and/or dairy products?
    a) Three or more
    b) Two
    c) One
    d) None

11) How many of your meals each day include raw fruit or vegetables?
    a) None
    b) One
    c) Two
    d) Three or more

12) Do you eat organic foods?
    a) Never deliberately
    b) Sometimes
    c) About 50 per cent of the food I eat is organic
    d) Always

13) Is your diet based on whole foods?
    a) No
    b) Some of my foods are unrefined
    c) Mostly
    d) Always

14) Do you add salt to your food, either at the table or when cooking?
    a) Always
    b) Often
    c) Sometimes
    d) Never

15) Are you overweight?
   a) Yes, by more than 7 kg/a stone
   b) Yes, but not more than 7 kg/a stone
   c) Yes, but not more than a few kilos/pounds
   d) No

For each A – score 0
For each B – score 1
For each C – score 2
For each D – score 3
Add up your score and match it with the evaluation below.

How did you score?

0–8
You need to look carefully at your lifestyle and focus on areas where you could improve. Can you cut back on alcohol for example, or cigarettes? Begin changes gradually but steadily and you will soon see real health benefits.

9–16
The degree to which you are destroying your health is equal to the degree you are creating it. By letting go of old unhealthy habits and developing new healthful practices you can tip the scales in your favour and experience the rewards of better health.

17–23
You are well on the way towards a healthy lifestyle, but there are still aspects that need changing if you are to experience a state of truly superior health. The time to begin living more healthfully is always now!

24–30
Congratulations, your current choices are creating a state of vibrant health for you. Remember, no matter how healthfully we live our lives there are always ways to improve, and new environmental and circumstantial challenges to rise to. Only by continuing to raise your awareness and develop your skills of healthful living can you be assured of a healthful future.

The Lifestyle Challenge

The challenge is simple: choose any aspects of your lifestyle to improve upon, so that by the end of 12 weeks you can honestly achieve an eight-point improvement in your score on this quiz. If you are already scoring 23 or above, then your goal is to achieve a score of 30. It's *that* simple *and* it's effective!

Chapter 2
A Time for Change

This chapter of the book offers a tour of the physical changes typical to the second half of our lives, and their implications for exercise and health. The majority of studies that have examined the changes that take place in the human body as it ages have been conducted on people living in the West. Very little is known about the physiological ageing of people who have lived a healthy and vigorously active lifestyle, consistently breathed clean air, and eaten a predominance of raw fruits and vegetables throughout their lives. In most texts on the subject of ageing, physical declines are largely bundled together with little or no differentiation being made between what is natural and what is caused by the accumulated effects of unhealthy living. This chapter focuses on those influences that appear to be exclusively age-related, as there are unquestionably certain changes that do result just from the passing of time. The good news is that these changes are generally only of major concern if you are attempting high levels of physical performance. It is nevertheless important to become familiar with how your body matures, so that you can make allowances where necessary and take action to minimize the rapidity with which you age.

The most influential factor in the ageing of the body is gradual dehydration. Human embryos begin life as about 90 per cent water. As the foetus grows, solid materials gradually replace some of the water. By the time an average person is in their forties, their body's water content is around 65 per cent, depending on the quantity of body fat they carry. The bodies of people over 80 may comprise less than 50 per cent water. This progressive dehydration partly occurs as an inevitable result of ageing, but diet and lifestyle are also a significant influence. One of the most relevant factors is a person's body composition. Muscle contains far more water than fat, about 70 per cent compared to less than 25 per cent. Therefore, maintaining activity and exercising regularly will help improve your muscle to fat ratio and your water content in turn, delaying the effects of dehydration.

Bones

Contrary to popular misconception, healthy bone density undergoes almost no change as people age, unless poor lifestyle and dietary choices have caused significant bone loss (osteoporosis). The hormonal changes that take place as a result of the menopause do *not* cause osteoporosis. If this were true, all post-menopausal women across the globe would show signs of osteoporosis by the time they were 60 – but they do not. In fact most of the world's female population, outside the West, maintain strong bones up until their death. At most, hormonal changes simply predispose a woman to being vulnerable to osteoporosis, should the causes of it be present, by slightly reducing her ability to absorb calcium. An unhealthy diet, smoking and inactivity are the main factors in the development of osteoporosis. (For more on the specific benefits of exercise, see Chapter 3).

Throughout your life, your bones have been continually undergoing the process of remodelling, old bone being reabsorbed and replaced with new. As you get older, there is a tendency for the rate of bone reabsorption to exceed the rate at which it is replaced. If you are eating and living healthfully, the difference will only be slight, and it can be easily counteracted by exercise and sufficient exposure to full spectrum sunlight.

Joints

In order to understand the changes that take place within your joints a little knowledge of your anatomy is necessary. All of your freely movable joints such as hips, elbows and knees, are encased in what are known as synovial capsules. These capsules are lined with a membrane that secretes synovial fluid into your joints. This fluid is vital, as it contains bone-feeding nutrients and keeps your joints lubricated. On each bone end, you have a shock-absorbent covering of fibrous tissue, called hyaline cartilage. Healthy cartilage is about 80 per cent saturated with synovial fluid and between 0.5 and 4 mm thick. Under pressure, as when you are standing for example, much of the synovial fluid is squeezed out of the cartilage, returning once the pressure is removed.

The tendency of your body to dehydrate as you get older can affect your joints by causing a reduction in the amount of synovial fluid produced and an increase in its viscosity (thickness). The more viscous your synovial fluid, the less readily it is absorbed by your cartilage. There is also a tendency for calcium from your joints to be deposited into the cartilage as you get older. This reduces the compressive and elastic qualities of the cartilage by causing it to become somewhat hard and brittle, making it less effective as a shock absorber.

Dehydration also affects your ligaments, the guy ropes that attach your bones to each other where they meet. Ligaments provide your joints with stability, and so are not designed to stretch. They do, however, have a quality of pliability that allows them to accommodate slight deviations from the joint's intended range of movement. As you grow older and your ligaments lose some of their water, they become less pliable and the more likely you are to sustain a sprain. Being aware of this, and ensuring that you warm up properly before undertaking vigorous exercise, provides powerful injury prevention.

The wear and tear on your joints that accumulates over the years also can result in a wearing down of the ends of your bones. As this occurs, you may progressively experience a feeling of stiffness in your joints when first rising in the morning or when you have been seated for an extended period. In otherwise healthy joints, this stiffness will quickly wear off once you start to move.

Muscles

In order to understand what happens to your muscles as you age, it's important first to understand how they work. The way that your muscles are put together resembles the construction of a Russian doll. The innermost and tiniest structures are called contractile proteins, which are contained within what are known as myofilaments. Bundles of myofilaments are then encased within larger tubes called myofibrils and bundles of myofibrils form the innards of your muscle fibres. Connective tissue is wrapped around all the individual parts of your muscles, holding them together and reducing friction between the different surfaces. The outermost layer of connective tissue wraps around the outside of the entire muscle and then extends at each end to form your tendons. The role of tendons is to provide an attachment between muscle and bone. As your muscles contract and pull on your bones, movement results.

The ability of a muscle to exert itself to the maximum in one massive effort (strength) is quite different from its ability to exert itself moderately but repeatedly (endurance). Lifting heavy suitcases into the back of the car is an example of muscular strength, whereas painting a ceiling requires endurance. When strength is combined with speed, the result is power.

Each of your muscles contains 'fast-twitch' fibres for performing strength and power work, and 'slow-twitch' fibres for performing endurance work. Within each muscle, you also have some fibres that are adaptable and can be trained for either strength or endurance tasks.

Strength work is anaerobic, meaning that oxygen is not needed by the muscle for it to work in this way. Your muscles are only able to endure repeated contractions, however, if oxygen is constantly delivered to them as they contract. This process is made possible by the presence of mitochondria, little fuel-making factories situated within your myofibrils. Carbohydrates and fats enter your mitochondria along with oxygen, where they are turned into fuel for endurance activities.

The primary by-product of strength work is lactic acid. This is what causes a burning sensation in your muscles when you perform intense work. Endurance work results in the production of carbon dioxide, water and heat.

Motor neurons are the pathways that allow for messages from your brain to be transmitted to your muscles. If you decide to pick something up from a table, your brain sends commands to the appropriate muscles of your shoulder, arm and hand, engaging them in the action. Muscles can only pull on bones; they cannot push them. When a muscle on one side of a joint contracts and pulls on the bones to bring about a movement, the one on the opposite side must lengthen to allow the movement to take place. In this way, muscles work in pairs. Flexibility is the ability of your muscles to stretch and accommodate large ranges of movement. When you experience a lack of flexibility, it is not usually your muscle fibres that are restricting you, but the connective tissue that is extensive throughout your muscles. Now that you have a basic understanding of the anatomy and terminology related to your muscles, let's look at what declines might occur as you get older.

Changes as You Age

Studies of older people have provided some insight into how muscular function typically declines with age. However, what is typical does not have to be inevitable. Many of the changes shown to occur during the second half of life are likely to have more to do with inactivity and poor dietary choices than with the passage of time.

Once over 50, a Westernized person typically loses about 1.5 per cent of their strength and 3.5 per cent of their power, per year. This seems to be due to various influences, including the death of a proportion of the motor neurones. When fewer messages are transmitted from the brain, there is a reduction in the number of muscle fibres that are activated. There also seems to be some reduced ability of the muscle fibres to grow (hypertrophy) in response to strength training. Declines in the nervous system are also the cause of slower reaction times and result in a reduced ability to move explosively (power). Once a motor neuron of any muscle fibre dies, the muscle fibre becomes dysfunctional. When this happens, the body in its wisdom extends a neighbouring neuron, from a nearby motor unit, to include and reactivate the fibre, which is called collateral innervation.

Although this is a marvellous thing as it helps to keep muscles fully functional, the result is a clumping of muscle fibres and a consequent loss of fine movement control and coordination. This collateral innervation of muscle fibres also has implications for endurance work, because there are more motor units involved in each movement. As a result, fatigue occurs sooner. A reduction in the size and number of fuel-making factories (mitochondria) has been shown to occur in older people. This reduces the ability of the muscle to endure extended periods of work. It is debatable whether or not this will occur to some degree even in people who exercise regularly. An overall reduction in the ability to regenerate fuel for muscular contraction is also a cause of reduced endurance potential and may partly be due to a lesser concentration of the enzymes needed for energy release.

As people get older they have less ability to tolerate lactic acid, the by-product of strength work, so they feel a burning sensation in their muscles sooner than a younger person does. The gradual dehydration that occurs with age also has an affect upon the muscle's connective tissue, making it less elastic and reducing its potential to be explosive. This loss of elasticity is more noticeable in terms of flexibility, and general stiffness that can be the first change people notice as they get older. The wonderful news is that flexibility can not only be maintained with appropriate stretching, but can actually be improved whatever a person's age.

Nervous System

It may surprise you to know that of all the aspects of physical functioning that decline with age, it is the nervous system that seems to be most affected. Although age-related changes are comparatively minimal, they are severely compounded by an unhealthy lifestyle and dietary habits. Because the nerves enable communication between the brain and the rest of the body, any decline in their function can have far-reaching effects on overall health.

The brain and spinal cord make up what is known as your central nervous system. You have 12 pairs of cranial nerves and 31 pairs of spinal nerves that extend out from your spinal cord. These nerves divide to form other nerves, which divide again thousands of times to reach every cell in your body. Your spinal nerves, and all the nerves that extend from them, make up your peripheral nervous system, consisting of two aspects: somatic and autonomic. Your somatic system connects your brain with your skeletal muscles and skin. Your autonomic system controls automatic processes such as digestive functioning and it has two opposing functions, sympathetic and parasympathetic. Your sympathetic function is responsible for speeding up actions such as constricting blood vessels, while your parasympathetic relaxes and diffuses activities. Neural communications rely on a low voltage electrical current for the transmission of messages. This electricity is conducted along neurons, which consist of dendrites that receive incoming information and an axon for transmitting outgoing messages. Axons are encased in a fatty substance known as myelin, which is a sheath that protects the nerve axon and allows for the quick transmission of messages. Throughout everyone's life, their brain cells are constantly dying, a process that increases with age. There are always an equal number of new nervous pathways awaiting development, however, but they will only come into play when stimulated to do so by demand. What this means is that the 'use it or lose it' motto applies as much to your brain as it does to your muscles. As people age, the death of nerve cells tends to accelerate. When coupled with a reduction in the brain's oxygen supply, this reduces the speed of incoming messages to the brain and slows the analysis of those messages once they arrive. The result is a reduced ability to balance and slower general reactions.

Due to what appears to be an age-related reduction in the efficiency of the sympathetic branch of the autonomic nervous system, there is a progressive decline in the ability to constrict blood vessels. This affects the adequate transport of blood and oxygen to the brain when rising quickly from lying or sitting. Typically, memory is reduced as people get significantly older. Usually events from long ago are remembered, while short-term memory is impaired. Oxygen deprivation to the brain is the prime culprit for this and this can also result in people finding it difficult to concentrate.

Losses in sight and hearing are common amongst older people, but not inevitable. For example, it is likely that older people will experience a gradual deterioration in their ability to hear high tones and sounds of speech. The fact that this is by no means true in all cases indicates that it is caused by factors other than ageing itself.

A progressive difficulty in focusing on things up close is also common. This is due to the lens of the eye losing its elasticity. The possible causes of this include the deposition (depositing of) of inorganic mineral salts, the accumulation of plaques in the microcirculation and age-related dehydration (see page 31). Another possibility is that a combination of dehydration and reduced efficiency of the muscles of the iris may lead to impairment of visual precision. The healthful functioning of most aspects of the nervous system is in some way related to the condition of the blood vessels. Reduced blood flow to the eyes, for example, causes the death of the photoreceptors and leads to vision impairment.

It is worth bearing in mind that as you get older there is a likelihood of your body awareness diminishing. This is partly due to changes in your nervous system, but primarily due to lack of performing the sort of dynamic and complex movements you did when you were younger. If your body awareness is poor, then be especially careful to achieve and maintain correct exercise technique. Lack of awareness is the forerunner to injury.

Heart and Lungs

By the time a person is aged 60, the sum total of changes affecting the heart, lungs and blood vessels typically causes a 25 per cent reduction in the oxygen supply to the cells of their body. Age-related declines actually play a very small part in these changes; rather it is inactivity and poor diet that are the main culprits. High blood pressure, heart disease, emphysema and stroke are all classic examples of conditions that are commonly associated with the second half of life, yet none of them are caused by the actual processes of ageing. These conditions are created exclusively by an accumulation of unhealthy diet and lifestyle habits. Some age-related changes do take place within the lungs, heart, and blood vessels, but these only affect athletic performance at the highest levels and do not affect moderate levels of exercise.

Before we move on to look at how ageing typically affects the respiratory system, we need to define a few respiratory-related terms. *Breathing rate* refers to how many times you complete a cycle of inhalation and exhalation in one minute. The term *residual volume* is used to describe the amount of air left in your lungs after you fully exhale. Your breathing rate and residual volume both contribute to your overall ability to take in, transport, deliver, and utilize oxygen (known as your V02 max). It also dictates how much carbon dioxide you can expel from your body.

Age-related Changes

The primary age-related changes that affect your breathing are dehydration and a consequent increase in the density of your tissues. These influences cause a reduction in the elasticity of the muscles positioned between your ribs (intercostals), your lungs and your alveoli, the tiny air sacs in the lung where the exchange of oxygen and carbon dioxide takes place. The effect of this, along with stiffening of the cartilaginous attachments between your ribs, is to restrict your chest in moving upwards and out-wards as you inhale. Compounding this there may be a loss in the capacity of your lungs to expand properly and fully inflate. Reduced elasticity of your alveoli also reduces your lungs' ability to take in air. The net result of these changes is shallower, faster, breathing and an increased residual volume. When you were a child, your residual volume was probably about 22 per cent, but by the age of 60 it may be 60 per cent. There is also a propensity for the development of fewer and larger alveoli as you get older. If this happens, an overall reduction in the surface area available for gaseous exchange will result.

The speed at which your heart contracts (beats) when you are at rest depends primarily upon its efficiency at pumping blood around your body. Although regularly raising your heart rate by vigorously exercising strengthens your heart, there comes a point of intensity where going beyond this may do your heart more harm than good. This is known as your maximum heart rate (MHR), and it is thought to decline with age. The reduction is probably due to a gradual decline in the efficiency of the part of your brain that controls nervous impulses. The standard way to calculate your MHR is to subtract your age from 220. The figure you end up with is the maximum number of times per minute your heart should beat.

Thermal Control

There does seem to be a tendency for older people to be more vulnerable to cold environmental temperatures. This has been identified as resulting from a combination of changes in the nervous system and a decrease in the skin density and the upper-most layer of fat (subcutaneous). This means that it is important to wear plenty of layers when exercising, particularly in cold environments.

Hormonal Changes

Just as the adolescent experiences shifts in hormonal activity, the older adult body undergoes changes within the endocrine system. In neither case are these natural occurrences manifestations of disease. Instead they are the natural evolution of the human organism as it experiences the passage of time. As both men and women grow older, their hormone-producing glands reduce the production of certain hormones. In healthy individuals, such changes produce few or no symptoms.

Male Hormonal Changes

Although much attention is paid to the 'change of life' in women, men undergo significant hormonal changes too. The two male hormones that are primarily involved are testosterone and aldosterone. As a man gets older, his levels of testosterone naturally drop. When this happens, there is a reduction in his potential to build muscle mass. As very few men ever develop their muscular potential, this reduction usually goes unnoticed. An older man whose work regularly demands heavy manual labour, or who performs callisthenics or weight trains, will have far greater muscular bulk than a sedentary man half his age.

A reduction in testosterone will also result in a slower metabolic rate, which can lead to a gain in body fat. This can be counteracted easily by regular exercise and good dietary habits. Another consequence of lowered testosterone production is a reduction in the red blood cell count. Aerobic exercise such as walking, swimming, or cycling, can offset this by increasing the amount of oxygen-carrying haemoglobin in the blood.

A man's libido may diminish as he gets older, but this certainly is not true for all men. The fast pace of living and the enervating recreational habits of younger people, along with the stresses of career pressures, often severely impairs sexual enjoyment. The potentially slower and more relaxed pace of later life can bring forth a whole new quality of lovemaking.

Hormones work in an intricate and interdependent way; the absence or presence of one affects the production of others. As testosterone levels fall, there is a consequent reduction in aldosterone. This hormone is responsible for promoting the retention of sodium, potassium and water by the kidneys. As aldosterone levels reduce, the ability to sweat when overheated is compromised. This means that heat stroke is more liable to occur when a person is vigorously active in hot climates, so extra care is needed to keep well hydrated. Aldosterone also helps the body to cope with stress, and its slow decline may be seen as an indication that nature assumes older men to be wiser and more peaceful. Any emotional difficulties experienced by men during their mid-life years probably have more to do with personal fears and expectations about getting older than are related to hormonal changes.

Female Hormonal Changes

The word menopause comes from the Greek words *meno* (month) and *pausis* (halt). It is used to describe the transition a woman's body undergoes as it naturally moves from its reproductive to non-reproductive state. Because every woman's biochemistry and physiology is unique, this gradual change can last anywhere from a few months to about fifteen years.

The two primary hormones involved in the female menopause are oestrogen and progesterone. Oestrogen is produced in the ovaries and stimulates growth, including that of breast tissue and the lining of the womb. Progesterone is produced by something called the corpus leuteum, a glandular mass formed in the ovaries following ovulation. The role of progesterone is to oppose oestrogen and keeps it in check.

Every month during the reproductive years of a woman's life, an egg follicle will ripen along with many others that only partially develop. The redundant non-mature eggs will go on to degenerate and be reabsorbed into the body. Each woman carries within her from birth only a certain number of eggs. By about the age of 45 there are few eggs left. As the number of available eggs diminishes they begin to mature irregularly. Gradually the ovaries slow down and eventually cease their production of oestrogen, as it is no longer needed for the maintenance of the reproductive system.

Although the ovaries of post-menopausal women no longer produce oestrogen, the liver, adrenal glands and fat cells continue to produce ample amounts of oestrogen to supply the rest of the body with its needs. It is progesterone that entirely disappears once ovulation ceases, because the corpus leuteum, its manufacturing plant, no longer forms once ovulation stops. Once progesterone is absent, oestrogen dominates and, if existing in unnaturally high levels its stimulating actions can lead to problems.

Nature does not intend for the level of oestrogen to get out of control once progesterone is no longer present. In fact, natural levels of oestrogen circulating the body of a healthy woman would not be dangerously high. This is exactly why progesterone would, under natural circumstances, no longer be required following menopause. The majority of women in the West, however, are not in a good state of health by the time they reach mid-life. This is primarily due to the accumulation of toxins that have entered their bodies over the years.

One specific group of toxins, known as xenoestrogens (meaning foreign oestrogens), can enter the body and act just like oestrogen. Post-menopausal women lack the presence of progesterone to keep oestrogen under control, resulting in xenoestrogens actively prompting the growth of reproductive structures, predisposing the body to cancerous developments of the breast and uterus. Xenoestrogens are found in pesticides, plastics, hair dyes, cosmetics, spermicides and drinking water. They come in their most concentrated form in dairy products and meat. This is due to the fact that farmed animals consume vast quantities of feed, grain and pasture that have been treated with a cocktail of chemical pesticides and fertilizers. The animals then store these toxins in their intramuscular fat and other adipose tissues.

In order to breeze through menopause, a woman needs to minimize the likelihood of unhealthily high levels of oestrogen. This is done by reducing the consumption of fat in the diet to healthy levels and avoiding animal products.

For her body to remain naturally balanced throughout menopause, a woman also needs an ample supply of vitamins and minerals. Vitamins C and E are especially important. A woman's body manufactures its own substance, known as PGE1, to calm any menopausal signs and symptoms. Ingredients for the PEG1 'recipe' include vitamins C, B3 and B6 as well as the two minerals zinc and magnesium. Animal fats have been shown to block the synthesis of PGE1 and are therefore best avoided.

In both men and women, there is a steady reduction in what is known as growth hormone (GH) as they get older. Although this results in a progressive loss of muscle tissue, the loss is minimal compared to the consequences of an inactive lifestyle.

The bottom line is that there are no purely age-related influences that can diminish your ability to achieve superior levels of fitness and health.

Chapter 3
The Power of Exercise

Physical activity is as vital to sustaining your life as the foods you eat. Try leaving your car parked in the garage for 20 years before taking it out for a drive. Even if the door does not fall off in your hand as you open it, the battery certainly won't turn the engine over. If you don't use it, you will lose it!

The older people become the less likely they are to be physically active. Yet a sedentary lifestyle contributes to premature ageing. With each advancing year, it becomes progressively more important to exercise. In our technologically driven Western society, with its labour-saving gadgets, moving walkways and cars, the human body is in grave danger of becoming redundant.

According to a national fitness survey conducted in the UK (Allied Dunbar, 1992), nearly one third of men and two thirds of women would find it difficult to sustain walking at a reasonable pace (3mph) up a 1 in 20 slope. The study also revealed that 30 per cent of men and 50 per cent of women aged 65 to 74 do not have sufficient muscle strength to lift 50 per cent of their body weight – and consequently have difficulty rising from a chair without using their arms.

The 1992 national fitness survey also revealed that while many people assume that their hectic lifestyle replaces the need to exercise, eight out of ten people do less exercise than is needed to benefit their health. This was surprising, because the report also documented that '80 per cent believe they do enough to keep fit'. This apparent lack of personal fitness awareness gives us partial insight into why such a low percentage of the population exercise. There is another key reason why inactivity is of epidemic proportions in the West, however, and this is a lack of education. Most people know that they 'should' exercise; yet they remain unmotivated to do so due to a lack of understanding the reasons why. Read on to fuel your enthusiasm to get up and move.

Physical fitness can be divided into five distinct areas (cardio-respiratory fitness, muscular strength, muscular endurance, flexibility and motor fitness) all of which, when trained, have a multitude of health benefits that can profoundly enhance the quality of your life.

Cardio-respiratory Fitness

Also known as aerobic fitness, cardio-respiratory fitness describes your body's efficiency at drawing in oxygen, transporting it to where it is needed and using it once it gets there. Your ability to do this depends primarily on the health of your heart, lungs and circulatory system. Having good cardio-respiratory fitness means that you will be better able to oxygenate the cells of your body and be more efficient at carrying toxic gasses and substances away from the cells. Both of these factors have extensive implications for your health, including massive reduction in your risk of cancer.

The passage of oxygen begins as you inhale. The amount you draw in with each breath depends upon various factors, including the ability of your air passageways (bronchus and bronchioles) and chest to fully expand, the strength and flexibility of your diaphragm and the elasticity of your lungs, as well as the viability of the alveoli within them. When you train your cardio-respiratory fitness, improvements will occur in all these areas. Your diaphragm and lungs will also receive a better blood supply as a result of changes in your heart and blood vessels.

Heart Anatomy

In order to appreciate fully the multitude of benefits that result from cardio-respiratory fitness, an understanding of some basic anatomy is required.

Your heart muscle is divided into right and left, with no direct communication between the two sides. Both sides are sub-divided into upper (atrium) and lower (ventricle) chambers. The right atrium receives blood that is carrying carbon dioxide. This blood then drops down into the right ventricle. From there it is sent on its way to be expelled from your lungs. The upper chamber of the left side is responsible for receiving oxygen-rich blood from the lungs. This blood is then dropped down into the left ventricle from where it is pumped under pressure out through the biggest artery in your body, the aorta. From the aorta, the oxygen-rich blood then travels through a whole network of arteries that deliver it throughout your body.

When you train your cardio-respiratory system, your left ventricle becomes a much stronger muscle. This means that each time your heart muscle contracts, it pushes a greater quantity of blood out through your aorta. This results in your heart needing to contract fewer times per minute in order to sufficiently oxygenate your body. It is not only your heart muscle that gets stronger with cardio-respiratory exercise; the walls of your arteries are also muscular, enabling them to pump blood along their lengths. With regular cardio-respiratory exercise, all your arteries will get stronger and therefore more efficient. The walls of your blood vessels will also become more flexible with this type of training. In the case of your arteries, it will reduce your risk of high blood pressure or aneurysm (rupturing of the artery wall when under pressure). In the case of your veins, this will reduce your risk of them becoming varicose.

Your veins are constructed in a different way from your arteries. Instead of having muscular walls to pump blood, they have a series of valves throughout their length. As blood migrates through each valve into the next section of the vein, the valve shuts behind it, preventing the backflow of blood. People who have poor cardio-respiratory fitness have a predisposition to weak valves. This results in some sections of the veins becoming engorged with back-flowing blood. When this happens, the veins become varicose – distorted, distended and unsightly.

The Importance of Oxygen

Because your heart is a muscle, it is vital that it continually receives its own supply of oxygen. This is made possible by what are known as coronary arteries, along with their accomplices, arterioles and the smaller capillaries. All of the improvements so far mentioned that relate to your blood vessels equally apply to the vessels that serve your heart. Having a fit cardio-respiratory system will therefore result in your heart itself being better oxygenated, healthier and more efficient. There is yet more good news as far as your heart is concerned. Your blood contains platelets, designed to enable it to clot should blood loss occur. It is partly the continual movement of your circulating blood that prevents it from clotting within your bloodstream. The more sedentary you become, the greater the likelihood that a thrombus (blood clot) may occur. Regular cardio-respiratory exercise promotes a dynamic flow of blood and so is a key factor in the prevention of thrombosis.

Blood Benefits

Cardio-respiratory fitness also has some very positive affects upon your blood. It increases the amount of haemoglobin you produce which, in turn, dictates how much oxygen you can attract across from your lungs into your bloodstream. If your circulatory system is fit, your blood is likely to maintain a healthier viscosity (thickness). Increased blood viscosity is another contributing factor to heart disease. This type of fitness training has also been shown to have a positive influence upon your cholesterol ratio, raising your desirable HDL carriers and reducing the undesirable LDLs.

If this is not enough to inspire you to rush out the door and get moving, the overall improvements that this aspect of fitness brings to your circulation will also result in you being less vulnerable to feeling the cold. Training your cardio-respiratory system can leave you laughing at British winters!

Muscular Strength

Muscular strength describes the ability of your muscles to push, pull, lift and carry significantly heavy objects. Having strong muscles carries with it many benefits, and every time you strengthen your muscles you are also strengthening your bones. Now that is a good deal!

Developing your strength will result in some increase in the size of your muscles. This is due to an increase in the contractile proteins deep within the muscle fibres. Women do not have the same capacity for increasing the size of their muscles as men do, because the development of muscle mass is heavily influenced by the presence of the hormone testosterone. For a woman to develop the size of her muscles naturally, to the degree seen amongst some female body builders, she would have to demonstrate a far greater dedication to strength training than most women are prepared to invest. A woman can, however, easily increase her strength to a point where she is considerably stronger than a sedentary man of her age.

The Benefits of Strength Training

By strengthening the muscles of your back and abdominals, you can go a long way to preventing back pain, and if you already suffer from back problems, increasing the strength of your torso can bring you much relief. Improvements in your posture, that can result from strength training, will also do a great amount to help any back problems you have. If being overweight is a challenge for you, strength training again comes to the rescue. Any increase in the amount of muscle mass you have on your body will have a positive effect on your metabolic rate. The greater your muscle mass, the faster your metabolic rate will be and, correspondingly, the easier it will be for you to burn off fat.

Strength training also increases the integrity your ligaments, which hold your joints in place, and your tendons, which attach your muscles to your bones. As a result, your joints become more stable and you are less likely to suffer from sprains, strains or tears. When your muscles are exerting their pure strength, oxygen is not involved in the breaking down of their fuel and lactic acid is produced as a result. The presence of lactic acid prevents your muscles from being able to continue to contract. With training, your muscles will become somewhat more resilient to the immobilizing affects of lactic acid. Consequently, they will be able to exert their strength for a slightly longer duration before becoming exhausted. For muscles to contract repeatedly for an extended duration, however, they must have good endurance.

Muscular Endurance

Muscular endurance is the stamina of your muscles. If you develop this aspect of your fitness, it will free you to enjoy a greater range of activities without fatiguing easily. This includes your sexual experiences.

Everyday tasks become easier to perform and far less tiring when you have good muscular stamina. This is made possible because this type of training results in two very significant improvements in your body. Firstly, it stimulates the growth of a more extensive capillary network to serve your muscles. This allows a lot more blood to be delivered to your slow-twitch fibres. (These are the types of fibres within your muscles responsible for all aerobic and endurance activities. They are red in colour and require a constant supply of oxygen if they are to contract.) Secondly, endurance training increases the size and number of your mitochondria (the fuel-making factories situated in amongst the myofibrils of your muscles). These two improvements result in your body being far more efficient at delivering oxygen to your muscles and utilizing it once it arrives.

Sustained good posture, which results in better health and appearance, is impossible to achieve without a significant degree of muscular endurance. Muscles with stamina are toned, and toned muscles contribute greatly to your appearance. Due to progressive dehydration, your muscles will have a tendency to increase in their viscosity as you get older, preventing them from contracting as smoothly. Regular participation in activities that challenge your endurance can almost entirely offset this. Regular endurance training will produce changes in your body's enzymes, making it easier for you to release stored body fat for use as fuel. This is a tremendous bonus if weight loss is one of your goals.

Flexibility

Flexibility describes the ability of your muscles to stretch, allowing for easy ranges of movement. Becoming flexible means that you can feel free to move your body as you desire without being restricted by tight muscles. It also means that you are less likely to become injured should you trip or fall. If you are flexible, you will be better able to achieve and sustain a good healthy posture. As a result, you will tire less quickly and be less vulnerable to back pain. The value of flexibility is typically underestimated in most fitness programmes. Once flexibility is lost, your quality of life will suffer greatly. In extreme cases of lost movement range, people may be unable to dress themselves, as is the case with many of our elders. When this occurs, it is easy to see how keeping flexible can make the difference between a life of independence and one of dependence upon others for the simplest tasks of everyday living. Muscular tightness can sneak up quickly as the years pass. Don't be caught out by postponing the development of a daily stretching habit. Chapter Five will show you how.

Motor Fitness

Motor fitness describes the efficiency of your nervous system, including its effects upon your balance, agility, reaction time, speed and coordination. All of these functions are vital to the quality of your everyday functioning. The natural processes of ageing have more impact upon these skills than any other aspect of your fitness. The good news is that by regularly participating in activities that challenge your motor fitness, you will be able to out-skill the average person your age. When it comes to reducing the likelihood of falling as you get older, nothing helps more than developing your motor fitness.

The combined rewards of all five components of fitness are more far-reaching than may first appear. There are certain subjects that are worthy of a special mention, as they are especially relevant for you as you get older.

Joints

Joints that can move within their fully intended range are far healthier than those that are stiff. When compromised in their ability to move, a series of events takes place within joints that can lead to their serious and permanent damage. Although the construction of joints was explained in the previous chapter, let's recap before continuing with this vitally important subject. A joint describes the junction of two bones. The ends of your bones that meet to form freely movable joints, such as elbows, hips and knees, are protected with a layer of cartilage. This cartilage protects the bone ends as they move against each other, acts as a shock absorber and is instrumental in transporting nutrients to the bone tissue.

Having a consistency similar to that of a sea sponge, the cartilage becomes relatively brittle, dense and non-yielding when dehydrated. Once engorged with synovial fluid, however, it transforms into a voluptuous cushion and effectively protects the bone ends. In order for the cartilage to remain hydrated, freely movable joints are encased in what is known as a synovial capsule. The membrane of this capsule, when stimulated to do so by movement, produces a fluid that keeps the cartilage lubricated. Joints that suffer from a lack of use produce little synovial fluid and, consequently, have dense, brittle and ineffective cartilage pads. Once dehydrated over an extended period of time, slits begin to appear in the cartilage, rather like the cracking of the earth during a drought. What little fluid there may be remaining inside leaks out, with the cartilage becoming even more desiccated.

Healthy joint cartilage does not contain nerve endings. Scar tissue, however, does. As the body attempts to repair its diseased joints, scar tissue is laid down and results in pain being felt on movement. This severely exacerbates the problem, as the individual is now even more hesitant to be active due to the pain experienced when doing so. Gradually a downward spiral of degeneration is occasioned, often to a point of losing physical independence. This state of disease is commonly referred to as osteoarthritis.

If your joints are not used to their full capacity over an extended period of time, they can become cripplingly painful and damaged beyond repair. By regularly partaking in activities that put your joints through their full ranges of movement and by performing daily the range of stretches set out in Chapter Five, you can ensure this does not happen to you.

Posture

The importance of good posture is greatly underestimated. At best, people acknowledge that it has an influence on the degree of back pain they suffer. Yet so much more than relieving back pain can be achieved in terms of improving your health and joy in living simply by working on this one aspect of your fitness.

Cardiorespiratory Benefits

Habitually holding your body in correct alignment will allow for free movement of your chest and diaphragm as you breathe. This means that with each inhale and exhale you will be breathing deeper, resulting in a greater intake of oxygen and a more efficient expulsion of carbon dioxide. When your body is not compressed by poor posture, your blood circulation will also improve. Having good circulation results in more than not suffering so much from the cold. Nutrients from the foods you eat, hormones produced from your endocrine glands, antibodies and waste products are all dependent upon your circulating blood for their transportation around your body. As your blood also transports oxygen and carbon dioxide, no amount of deep breathing will meet the needs of your cell's respiration if your circulation is sluggish.

Improved Immune Functioning

Having a body that is poised and graceful will enhance the flow of your lymphatic fluids and consequently improve your immune functioning. You will be better at getting rid of toxic wastes and activating your defences. Improving your ability to exhale carbon dioxide and rid yourself of such waste will reduce the acidity of your blood. An overly acid bloodstream is an underlying contributory cause of most conditions of ill health and the primary cause of osteoporosis. When this is understood, it can be appreciated that developing good posture is a key to maintaining a healthy bone density.

Digestive Relief

It is common for people who have suffered from years of digestive problems to find instant relief by simply adopting a superior posture. When held in proper alignment, your intestinal tract is able to function unimpeded and the foods you eat will be digested, absorbed, taken up into your blood, and utilized with far greater ease and efficiency. Believe it or not, poor posture can be a cause of malnutrition.

Joint Health

Your posture not only affects your internal organs and processes – it has tremendous influence upon the health of your joints. If your posture is poor, your joints will not be held and used in correct anatomical alignment. This means that some aspects of your joint surfaces will be placed under tremendous pressure while other areas will make little or no contact with adjoining bones. The result is an uneven wear of your joint surfaces, with certain areas subjected to excessive stress, causing the breakdown of your protective cartilage. The consequence is a gradual and progressive deterioration of your joints. The superior posture you adopt today will contribute greatly to a healthy and pain-free future for your joints. A compromised posture will impede the mechanical functioning of your muscles, resulting in reduced ranges of strength and loss of flexibility. Your muscles will function far more effectively when supported by correct alignment of your bones.

Spine Health

Perhaps the most serious implication of poor posture is the effect it has upon the alignment of your spine. This is not only because incorrect spinal alignment has an extensive negative impact upon everything mentioned so far, but also because it will impede the functioning of your nervous system. When your spine is misaligned, especially at your cervical area (neck), it impinges upon the nerves that extend from your spinal cord. As every cell in your body is dependent upon efficient communication with your brain via your nervous system pathways, this has very serious implications indeed. It is for this reason that a collapsed or distorted posture can impact upon the health of every cell, tissue, organ and system in your body.

Compaction of cervical vertebrae also reduces the oxygen supply to your brain and eyes. This results in problems with eyesight, slower mental processing and reduced clarity of thought. Correcting the alignment of your spine can enhance even your senses of smell, taste and hearing. The combination of increased oxygen to your head and reduced impaction of your cervical vertebrae will result in far fewer headaches.

Improving Your Posture

As we get older, there is a tendency for us to allow our bodies to undergo what can be compared to a landslide. There is, in most cases, absolutely no need for this to occur. Poor posture supports a disempowered and negative mental attitude that, in turn, creates a worsening posture. To lift yourself out of this escalating rut, all you need to do is to correct the way you hold your body when sitting, standing and walking. Better posture goes a long way to improving your appearance, and this can have a very positive affect on your self-esteem. By improving your posture, you can significantly improve your health on almost every level.

Below are some typical incorrect postural habits that people develop when sitting, walking and standing. Study the illustrations depicting the correct way to do these things and then practise them whenever you can throughout your day. If you spend extended periods of time sitting or standing, it is likely that you will gradually sink into poor posture. To avoid this happening, make a point of taking a break every 20–30 minutes to realign your posture.

As you can see in Figure 3.1, your spine is not designed to be straight like a rod. It has natural curves, primarily for the purpose of dispersing shock. Attempting to remove these natural curves not only places the rest of your body in an unnatural position, but also results in your brain receiving more shock waves than it

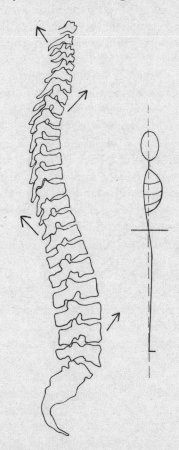

Figure 3.1 The spine

is designed to accommodate as you walk, run or play. Problems occur when a lack of muscular control allows these curves to become exaggerated and excessive.

An exaggerated curve in the lower back (often seen in pregnant women and men with beer bellies) compacts the lumbar vertebrae and is a common cause of back pain.

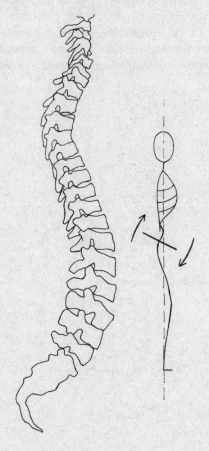

Figure 3.2 *Curve in lower back*

An exaggerated curve in the upper back (often seen in office workers and potters) compacts the breathing and internal organs.

An exaggerated curve in the cervical vertebrae will restrict blood flow to everything above it, including the brain and eyes, and interfere with the functioning of the nervous system.

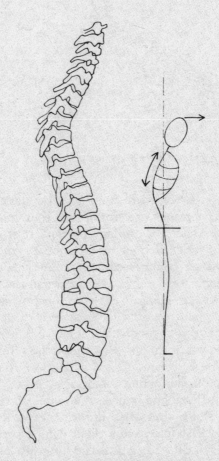

Figure 3.3 *Exaggerated curve in upper back*

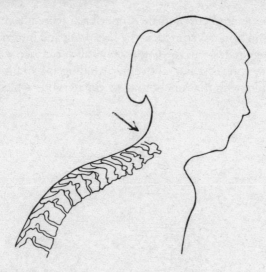

Figure 3.4 *Exaggerated curve in cervical vertebrae*

There is a tendency when sitting to allow the chest to drop downwards. This results in a need to lift your chin in order to look straight ahead of you causing a pinching of the vertebrae in your neck. The result of poor sitting posture is that all of your internal organs are compressed, compromising their function. The blood supply to your eyes, nose, ears and taste buds is also impeded. If you are going to eat your lunch while working at your computer (not recommended), at least sit up properly so that you can taste your food and see the computer screen. The acute angle at which this poor posture places your neck also compromises your neural pathways and so has a negative influence on the healthful functioning of every cell of your body.

The weight of your body when sitting should be taken by your sitting bones, which are located in the centre of each buttock. Your lower back should have a slight natural curve, and your sternum (breast bone) should be facing forwards. Your shoulders should be relaxed down and slightly back, and your neck long.

As you can see, it is vital for good posture to have the height of your chair and desk correct for you. A desk that is too low in relation to your chair will encourage the incorrect posture described above.

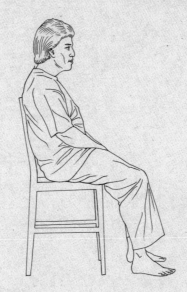

Figure 3.5 *Sitting (Incorrect)*

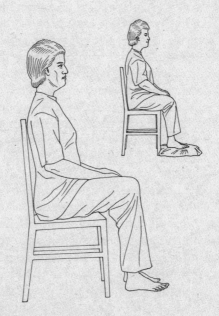

Figure 3.6 *Sitting (Correct)*

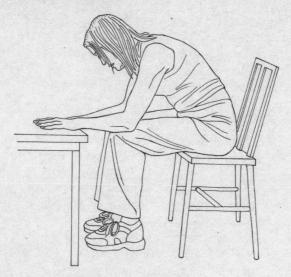

Figure 3.7 *Incorrect Chair/Desk Height Ratio*

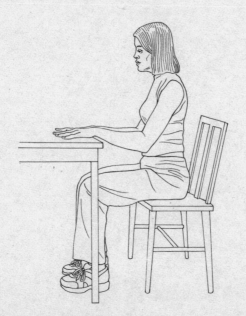

Figure 3.8 *Correct Chair/Desk Height Ratio*

Cushions and/or large books can be used to correct your chair/desk height ratio.

When standing, especially for long periods of time, there is a tendency to place more weight on one leg than the other. This places an uneven stress on your pelvis, reduces blood flow and sets you up for postural misalignment throughout the rest of your body. When one hip is dropped, the pelvis is tilted at an angle, resulting in your spine being thrown, laterally, out of alignment. There can be a tendency for an exaggerated curve to develop in the lower back when standing; stooping with shoulders rounded and the pubic bone thrust forwards is another example of poor posture.

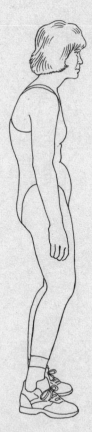

Figure 3.9 *Standing (Incorrect)*

Your weight should be distributed equally on both feet. Your knees should be straight but not locked. There should be only natural curves throughout the spine. Your shoulders need to be relaxed down and slightly back, and your neck should be long.

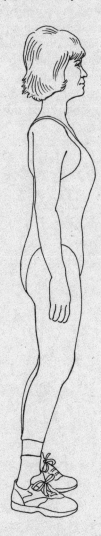

Figure 3.10 *Standing (Correct)*

The most likely thing to cause poor posture when walking is looking down at the ground, as doing so tips the whole body forward. Although looking where you are going is necessary, try to walk with your chin parallel to the ground and use your eyes to look downwards a few feet in front of you.

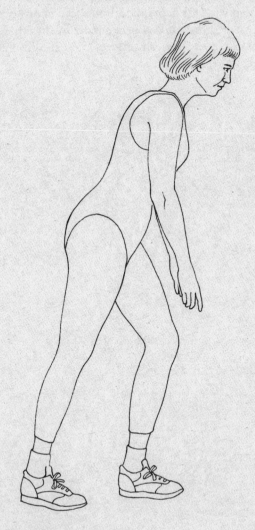

Figure 3.11 *Walking (Incorrect)*

Elegant walking requires a mindset of grace. The outer portion of the heel should strike the ground first and then a rolling action through the foot should propel you forwards from the inner portion of the ball. The arms should swing naturally by the sides and the head should be held high, but not tipped back. Being light on your feet begins with a good night's sleep and a positive outlook. Tiredness and depression both have enormous negative influences on posture and, consequently, on health. This is an excellent example of how all aspects of a healthy lifestyle are interdependent.

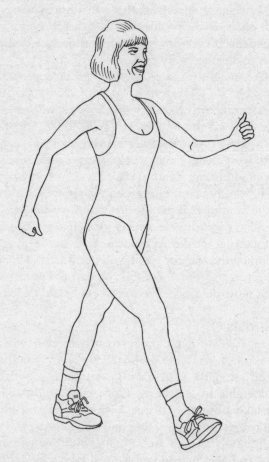

Figure 3.12 *Walking (Correct)*

Weight Control

The age-related reasons why people are more likely to gain weight as they grow older could be written on a postage stamp. By far the greatest causes are a poor diet and insufficient exercise. If diet alone is addressed and no attention paid to exercise, weight loss can be frustratingly slow or not occur at all. When considering the type of exercise most useful for fat loss, it needs to be understood that fat can only be broken down for use as fuel if oxygen is present. For this reason, cardio-respiratory (aerobic) exercise and activities involving muscular endurance are the best fat burners. Muscular endurance training also brings about positive changes in your enzyme profile, meaning that there is a reduction in your tendency to lay down fat and an increased efficiency in your ability to liberate fat for fuel.

Muscular strength training also has a very important role in weight loss, but for a different reason. As mentioned above, the more muscle you have on your body, the faster will be your metabolic rate. This results in a more rapid utilization of calories 24 hours a day. Finally, if you are overweight, remember that postural improvements can also help because they can reduce the load on your joints and create a more slender impression.

As far as your health is concerned, being overweight is undesirable from any angle. It predisposes you to a plethora of problems including heart disease, cancer, diabetes, arthritis and back pain. By following the dietary guidelines set out in Chapter One, and developing the exercise habit, you can watch the pounds fall away and reveal the more youthful you that is awaiting your discovery. For more detailed advice on obesity, see Chapter Six.

Osteoporosis

Osteoporosis is the name given to a condition whereby demineralization of the bone tissue takes place, causing it to lose density and strength. Osteoporosis results in bones that are highly vulnerable to fracturing. Once in this diseased state, it may only take a bumpy car ride to break ribs or a trip on the pavement to fracture a hip. This condition affects both men and women, although women are at higher risk due to having less bone mass to begin with. Here we will take a look at the vital role of exercise in keeping bones healthy and strong.

There are two types of cells related to bone metabolism: osteoblasts, which create new bone, and osteoclasts, which break down old bone. In a healthy adult, both types of cells are equally active, resulting in bone constantly being renewed and replaced. In the Western world, by the time a woman is age 30, the activity of her osteoclasts begins to outstrip that of her osteoblasts. The result is a gradual and progressive loss of bone density and bone mass.

Two types of exercise that are the most effective in stimulating osteoclast activity are those involving skeletal impact and those requiring muscular strength. The shock waves that travel up through your body as you walk briskly are sufficient to stimulate the activity of your bone-building cells. This type of exercise will only serve to strengthen the bones of your legs, pelvis and lower back, because the shock waves are largely dispersed by the time they reach your midline. In Chapter Six, you will be introduced to a variety of exercises for stimulating bone growth in your upper body. Strength work is also a bone-building activity, because every time your muscles contract, they pull on your bones via your tendons. This challenges the bones to stay strong in order to cope with the force exerted by the tendons. Having strong muscles provides your bones with stability and so reduces the likelihood of them becoming damaged should you fall. Strength training also increases the integrity of your ligaments, which is vital for maintaining correct alignment of your joints.

Although during vigorous exercise your blood becomes temporarily more acidic, the long-term result of regular physical activity is increased blood alkalinity. As overly acidic blood is the cause of osteoporosis, exercise is of tremendous benefit.

Your Pelvic Floor

Your pelvic floor is a hammock of muscle that is suspended between your pubic bones and tailbone. Its job is to help retain and support your internal organs by counteracting the downward pull of gravity. The muscles of the pelvic floor are also involved in urination, defecation and sexual intercourse.

Both the male and female anatomies have pelvic floors, with only minimal differences in their design. The female has three openings in its structure, the urethra, vagina and anus. The male pelvic floor has only two: the urethra and anus. The female is therefore more vulnerable to damaging this muscle. If the pelvic floor becomes weak, it has implications for bladder and anal continence as well as sexual pleasure. A weak pelvic floor has poor blood circulation and lymphatic flow. This results in an increased risk of infections and other problems of the genital tissues. As the pelvic floor is attached to the front and back of your pelvis, it also plays an important role in stabilizing your pelvis. In conjunction with the development of strong abdominal muscles, exercising the pelvic floor can help to relieve lower back and sciatic pain.

Exercising Your Pelvic Floor Muscle

In order to exercise your pelvic floor, you first need to locate it. The following applies equally to men and women. Sit on a chair with your legs slightly apart and relax your tummy muscles. Clench your buttocks and release them a few times. Become familiar with this feeling and know that *this is not the pelvic floor*. Now relax the buttocks and pull your tummy in tight a few times. Become familiar with this feeling and know that *this is also not the pelvic floor*. Now, relax your tummy and buttocks and squeeze your thighs together a few times. Become familiar with this feeling and know that *this is not the pelvic floor either*. Now that you are familiar with what it is *not*, you can go on to find it and isolate it.

Remain in your chair with your legs relaxed and slightly apart. Release any tension from your tummy muscles, legs and buttocks. Now imagine that you need to urinate, but that it is not convenient to do so. Contract the muscles you would need to contract in order to withhold urine. Be sure that your tummy, buttocks and legs remain relaxed as you do it. Release and repeat. A good way to find out if you have located the muscles correctly is to stop the flow of urine for a moment, mid-stream, next time you go to the toilet. If you are able to do so, you have successfully located the pelvic floor. Although this is an effective way to ensure you have the right muscle, it is not advisable to practise this method habitually, as it can cause a back flow of urine and lead to infections.

When to Exercise

An excellent time to exercise your pelvic floor is every time you go to pick up anything that would be too heavy for you to lift with one finger. Contract your pelvic floor first, followed by your tummy muscles, by pulling your belly button towards your spine. This will not only ensure these muscles get regularly exercised, but it will go a long way toward preventing back pain. Standing in a queue provides another opportunity for this type of exercise. Simply stand with your legs slightly apart and repeatedly contract your pelvic floor muscles. Developing the habit of exercising this important area when doing certain habitual tasks, such as cleaning your teeth or washing up, can ensure that you remember to include them in your day.

Muscles are made up of some fibres that are designed to endure long steady bouts of repeated contraction (slow twitch); other fibres are designed for instant and intense contractions of short duration (fast twitch). It is the endurance (slow twitch) fibres of the pelvic floor that support your undercarriage as you go about your daily tasks. There are times, however, when the power (fast-twitch) fibres need to come into play, such as when you trip or jump. On these occasions, the muscles are required to make a quick snatching action in order to support the pelvic contents. This means that when exercising the pelvic floor, it is valuable to incorporate both fast and slow contractions.

Once you have located the pelvic floor and mastered simple contractions, you can go on to work more specifically for even greater tone and control. Experiment with the following variations:

1. Pull up the muscles from the back (anus) and then gradually bring the contraction around to the front (urethra).
2. Reverse the above by starting at the front and moving towards the anus.
3. Pull up the entire pelvic floor in stages, as if going up in a lift, and then lower it back down.
4. Make a pumping action with the entire pelvic floor.
5. Progress all of the above by widening your stance while you perform the exercises.

Strengthening your pelvic floor not only maintains, or re-establishes, continence, it also increases your sexual enjoyment, improves the general health of your genital area and is vital in the prevention of prolapses. If you feel shy about exercising in front of other people, then exercising your pelvic floor is a good one for you. No one will know you are training your pelvic floor unless you raise your eyebrows as you do it!

Safety

As you get older, safety becomes more worthy of concern, in that if you do get injured, it typically takes longer for you to heal than when you were younger. There are two potential ways to get hurt: by injuring yourself; by being injured by someone or something else. The latter, commonly referred to as personal safety, is sadly an issue for everyone. The advancing years can leave you feeling more vulnerable to injury from others. Achieving and maintaining a good level of fitness, however, can help overcome these fears. Allaying fears is important, as a feeling of vulnerability acts as a magnet for aggressors.

Training your reactions by participating in activities and games such as racket sports will make a valuable contribution to your personal safety. Muscular strength training will also result in your having quicker reactions, in addition to your becoming more physically capable of protecting yourself. In the distant past, it was common for our ancestors to need to escape from a predator. In modern times, any threat is usually from other humans. In either case, a good level of aerobic fitness can make the difference between escape and injury.

Energy

There is no reason for tiredness to be part of the second half of your life: old is not synonymous with tired. Tiredness occurs when the workload of your body exceeds the capacity of your nervous system to coordinate it. When this occurs, the way to overcome it is to reduce your body's workload and recharge your nervous system with increased sleep. One of the greatest enemies of fatigue is stimulation, in that any form of it will increase your body's workload. The cup of coffee you drink to 'get you going' may jolt you into overcoming your tiredness in the morning, but your body will exert its nervous vitality for the rest of the day in an attempt to rid the poisons from your body. The result is that the next morning you feel even more exhausted and so need even more coffee to get you going.

Another enemy of tiredness is lethargy. In addition, every time you are physically active, you are helping to keep your lymphatic fluids flowing. Unlike your blood, your lymphatic fluids are not pumped around your body by a heart muscle. Lymphatic flow relies instead on changes in pressure, as brought about by exercise, to keep it mobile. Insufficient physical movement results in sluggish lymphatic processing and a consequent accumulation of toxins. The more toxic your body, the greater its workload and the more predisposed you are to experiencing fatigue. A lack of exercise can also be the cause of poor food choices as lethargy seeks stimulation.

For numerous reasons, including its effectiveness in reducing stress, exercise provides one of the best cures for insomnia. There is another rather fascinating reason too. In order for your body to be triggered into its sleeping mode, it requires a slight drop in its internal temperature. Typically, there is a drop in internal temperature about five hours following a significant intensity and duration of physical exertion. If you participate in vigorous activity about five hours before attempting to sleep, you are more likely to drift off into dreamland easily.

Psychological Health

Exercise is famous for being useful in the management of stress. Your body is programmed to assume that any anxiety you feel results from a physical threat to your life. As a consequence, when anxiety of any form arises, your body prepares itself for fighting or running. This involves a chain of physiological events initiated by your nervous system and includes changes in the production and activity of your hormones and shifts in the distribution of your blood. Once in this state of high physiological arousal, if you exercise vigorously, your bodily processes soon return to normal. If, however, you remain sedentary, the effects of the fight or flight response accumulate and contribute to causing a host of health problems.

Being regularly physically active will also enable you to better manage feelings of anger and frustration, as it will provide you with a physical outlet for these self-destructive states. Going for a long walk, run, or cycle can be a form of meditation, providing you with the mental space to gain a more peaceful and healthy perspective on life. As we get older, there is potentially a loss in our physical grace, which can leave us with a poor self-image and, consequently, reduced self-esteem. There is no reason, however, that you should lose your physical beauty as you get older. A well cared for old car is considered a valuable vintage item. On the other hand, an old car that has been neglected is generally viewed as fit only for the scrap heap. One woman was quoted as saying that she had married an anthropologist knowing that the older she got the more he would appreciate her!

It is with that in mind that I offer you my wholehearted encouragement and support to walk, run, jump, skip, pull, push, reach, stretch and lift your way to a beautiful older body and a vibrantly healthy physique.

How Fit are You?
Now is your chance to evaluate your current fitness.

1) Do you partake in sustained activities that cause your breathing rate and pulse to significantly increase (such as brisk walking, cycling, swimming, or dancing) for a minimum of 30 minutes?
   a) Less than once a week
   b) Once or twice a week
   c) Three or four times a week
   d) Five times a week or more

2) Do you partake in activities that challenge your physical strength (such as weight training or heavy manual labour)?
   a) Less than once a week
   b) Once or twice a week
   c) Two to three times a week
   d) Four times a week or more

3) Do you perform tasks, sports or other activities that challenge the ability of your muscles to work for extended periods of time (such as washing windows, moderately heavy gardening, rowing, playing tennis, interior decorating or hiking)?

    a) Less than once a week
    b) Once or twice a week
    c) Three or four times a week
    d) Five times a week or more

4) Do you stretch your muscles either by doing yoga or other specific forms of stretching?
    a) Less than once a week
    b) Once or twice a week
    c) Three to five times a week
    d) Six to seven times a week

5) Do you participate in activities and/or sports that challenge your reaction times (such as racket sports or exercise to music classes)?
    a) Less than once a week
    b) Once or twice a week
    c) Three or four times a week
    d) Five times a week or more

6) Do you participate in activities and/or sports that challenge your coordination (such as dancing or racket sports)?
    a) No
    b) Not generally
    c) Sometimes
    d) Regularly

7) Do you participate in activities that challenge your balance (such as yoga, dancing, martial arts, water-skiing, ice-skating or gymnastics)?
    a) Less than once a week
    b) Once or twice a week
    c) Three or four times a week
    d) Five times a week or more

8) How is your posture?
   a) Poor
   b) It could be improved upon
   c) Reasonably good
   d) Excellent

9) Do you walk, jog, run, cycle, or skate rather than take the car?
   a) Rarely or never
   b) Occasionally
   c) Frequently
   d) Always, if possible

10) Can you get down on to the floor and back up again without using your arms?
   a) No
   b) Almost
   c) Yes, with great effort
   d) Yes, easily

For each A – score 0
For each B – score 1
For each C – score 2
For each D – score 3

Add up your score and match it with the evaluation below:

How did you score?

0–8

You are leading a sedentary lifestyle and, consequently, you will age prematurely. Due to your inactivity, you are also increasing the risk of various conditions of compromised health. The good news is that fitness can always be developed and the physical deterioration that results from being sedentary can, generally, be reversed. By undertaking The Fitness Challenge, as outlined in Chapter Five, you can gradually regain both your physical functioning and your youthfulness.

9–16

Being busy is not the same as being active. Although your lifestyle is not totally sedentary, your level of physical activity is far below that needed for health and longevity. Before you reap the consequences of your lost fitness, take action by undertaking The Fitness Challenge as outlined in Chapter Five.

17–23

You are more active than the majority of people in the West. If your goal is vibrant health, youthfulness and longevity, then there is a need for you to make an even greater commitment to your physical fitness. The Fitness Challenge, described in Chapter Five, provides you with a progressive way to build your aerobic fitness, muscular strength, muscular endurance and flexibility.

24–30

You are an athlete and being so will reap great dividends in terms of your health, youthfulness and longevity. Training those areas of your fitness that are least developed is the best way forward. The Fitness Challenge in Chapter Five will help to ensure that your fitness is comprehensive by guiding you in the identification of your strengths and weaknesses.

Chapter 4
Preparing to Exercise

The Principles of Fitness Training

One of the wonderful things about your body is its willingness, readiness and ability to bring about changes within itself in response to challenging influences. Fitness training is based on this same ability of your body to adapt when challenged. Applying an appropriate degree of challenge, and sufficient recovery, is the key to effective fitness training. If the challenge is too great, or recovery insufficient, then injury or gradual breakdown of your body on some level is the predictable outcome. If the challenge is too slight, then it will not bring about any improvements in your body's abilities. The term *overload* is used to describe the correct intensity of physical challenge needed to bring about positive improvements in your fitness, known as the *training effect*.

The dividing line between overload and *overwork* (excessive challenge) becomes finer as you age. It is vital – if injuries are to be avoided and potential benefits fully realized – that you remain aware of this distinction as the years go by. The feasible challenges of overload that result in a positive training effect can easily become the unrealistic expectations of overwork that lead to injury. It is also worth noting that as you advance in years, any temporary discontinuation of exercise, for whatever reason, will tend to result in a more rapid loss of fitness. This means that if you become ill, or for any reason remain sedentary for several days in a row, when you return to your fitness pursuits you need to spend time re-establishing your previous fitness levels before continuing.

Goal Setting and Progressing

The first step in preparing to exercise involves the identification of your fitness goals. Now that you have an understanding of the five components of physical fitness, it is possible for you to be more specific in this endeavour. The classic declaration, that 'this year I am going to get fit,' typically made by people on the first of January every year, is far too general to be of any practical use. The appropriate reply to such a statement is 'fit for what?'

If you are serious about wanting to improve your fitness, then it will serve you to begin by considering your long-term goals. Do you want to maintain your current level of fitness in the years to come? Do you want to substantially improve your fitness? Might you have aspirations to compete athletically or achieve exceptionally high standards of athleticism? If maintaining your current fitness is all that you desire, then you need to measure how fit you currently are so that you will have something to compare yourself with in the future. This is also true if you want to improve your fitness substantially. You need a reference point.

To have a high level of athletic performance as your goal, you will need to become clear what constitutes having achieved that. Perhaps it is winning a certain competition or, if you are not competitive, achieving a certain feat.

For goals to be effective they need to be SMART – specific, measurable, achievable, revisable and time oriented. To have a goal that one day you will be fit is of no value. As your body ages, it will probably respond to training at a slower rate than it did when you were younger. Progress will still occur, but improvements might take a little longer to become apparent. For this reason, it is especially important that you break your long-term goals down into shorter-term segments. This will ensure that your achievements are identified and that your motivation is upheld.

This book presents a 12-week programme of fitness training, offering four levels of progression. It is recommended that you use this only as a time guide. Your body may have a different agenda and so it may take you 24 or even 36 weeks to achieve the next level. If this happens, focus on listening to your body and working with it, rather than feeling despondent. Slower responses to fitness training can occur for numerous reasons, most of which are to do with one or more unhealthful aspects of diet or lifestyle. If you are not getting the results you hope for, then revisiting Chapter One is a good idea.

Unless you have some specific physical limitations, you can begin at Level 1 and eventually achieve all of the exercises in

Level 4. Let's take a look at the five fitness components and consider what your goals might be.

Goal Setting and Measuring the Progress of Your Aerobic Fitness

There are many ways that you can evaluate your aerobic fitness without involving expensive or intimidating equipment. One way is to take your pulse first thing in the morning before getting out of bed. This will be a measurement of what is called your resting heart rate. In the absence of other influences such as drugs, coffee or stress, the more aerobically fit you are, the slower will be your resting heart rate. This is because a fit heart is a strong one that can process a lot of blood with each contraction and therefore needs to contract less often. If your aerobic goal is to maintain your current fitness level, you need to establish your current resting heart rate and then check it monthly to see if it has remained the same. If your goal is to be substantially fitter than you currently are, then a six-point decrease in your heart rate, over a period of three months, would be a realistic goal.

Another simple way to evaluate the effectiveness of your aerobic training is by measuring your aerobic achievements. This is especially useful if partaking in a competition is your goal. The way to do this is to measure a specific distance and then time how long it takes you to cover it. This can be applied equally to walking, running, cycling or swimming, all of which are predominantly aerobic activities. If 12 weeks from now you can cover a predetermined distance in the same amount of time as you can today, then you are being successful in maintaining your aerobic capacity. If after 12 weeks training you can cover a specified distance 20 per cent quicker, this will qualify as a substantial improvement.

Goal Setting and Measuring the Progress of Your Muscular Strength

When it comes to muscular strength, the same basic principles apply. First you need to ascertain your current strength. All training is very specific. Your body will make positive adaptations directly according to the ways in which you challenge it. For example, the strength and flexibility of a tennis player's serving arm provides no guarantee that she or he has what it takes to deliver a powerful golf swing. Just because a person can walk for mile upon mile without tiring does not mean that they can tread grapes with the same stamina. This aspect of physical fitness training is known as the law of specificity, and it applies as much to muscular strength as to all of the other fitness components. If you are just starting out on the fitness path, it is helpful for you to evaluate the strength of your upper and lower body separately. This is because you have probably developed your current level of strength according to your occupation and lifestyle. If you are a doting parent or grand-parent, your arms are possibly stronger than your legs as a result of picking up and carrying small children. Perhaps you enjoy hiking in the hills and have visible leg muscles to show for it, but do little to challenge the strength of your arm muscles.

By trying the following exercises to evaluate your strength, you will be able to identify which level of the strength programme offered in Chapter Five is appropriate for you to begin with. These tests, and the ones that follow for endurance, are limited in the sense that they only provide you with a way to measure the strength and endurance of a limited number of muscle groups. When you come to the exercise programme in Chapter Five, it will explain how you can use the programme to design your own personalized training regimen. If your goal is to maintain your current degree of muscular strength, then evaluating your success is easily achieved by taking note of which exercises you can perform and the number of sets you can achieve. Then simply test yourself every month by repeating the same strength chal-lenge and assessing if you can still do it. After 12 weeks, an ability to perform the strength exercises one level up (see Chapter Five) or to perform twice the number of sets (groups of repetitions), demonstrates a substantial improvement in your strength. If your goals exceed this and you want to achieve levels of strength greater than those in the programme, then it is worthwhile invest-ing in the advice of a qualified fitness consultant.

NB: Using appearance as a way of measuring your muscular strength or endurance is not an accurate evaluation. Apart from being very subjective, the gain or loss of body fat can be deceiv-ing. Even small reductions in body fat will reveal underlying muscles, giving the impression that the muscles themselves have grown or increased in tone, which may or may not be the case.

Assessing the Strength of Your Lower Body

1. Can you get up out of an easy chair without using your arms
   either to push on the chair or to push on your own thighs? If
   not, most of the exercises in Level 1 of the lower body
   strength programme will suit you to start with.
2. Can you get up out of an easy chair without using your arms
   while holding something weighing 3 lb? If not, most of the
   exercises in Level 2 of the lower body strength programme
   will suit you to start with.
3. Can you get up out of an easy chair without using your arms
   while holding something weighing 5 lb? If not, most of the
   exercises in Level 3 of the lower body strength programme
   will suit you to start with.
4. Can you get up out of an easy chair without using your arms
   and standing up on only one leg? If not, most of the exercises
   in Level 4 of the lower body strength programme will suit you
   to start with.

If you can achieve this already, then work with Level 4 of the
upper body strength programme, but perform six sets instead of
four and/or increase the weight of any dumbbells you use to do
the exercise.

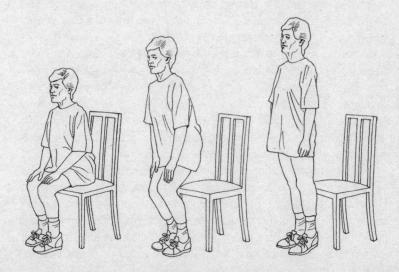

Assessing the Strength of Your Upper Body

1. Can you perform three box push-ups (see below)? If not, most of the exercises in Level 1 of the upper body strength programme will suit you to start with.
2. Can you perform three extended box push-ups? If not, most of the exercises in Level 2 of the upper body strength programme will suit you to start with.
3. Can you perform three modified push-ups? If not, most of the exercises in Level 3 of the upper body strength programme will suit you to start with.
4. Can you perform three full push-ups? If not, most of the exercises in Level 4 of the upper body strength programme will suit you to start with.

If you can already achieve this, then work with Level 4 of the lower body strength programme, but perform six sets instead of four and/or increase the weight of any dumbbells used to do the exercise.

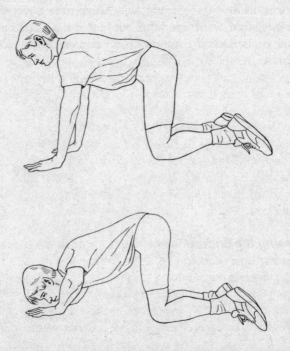

Goal Setting and Measuring the Progress of Your Muscular Endurance

Your aerobic fitness achievements can provide you with considerable insight into the ability of your muscles to endure. In order to sustain the movements necessary to challenge your heart, lungs, and blood vessels, you need to repeatedly contract muscles. If you can walk or jog several miles with ease, it is proof that your leg muscles have admirable endurance. In order to swim several lengths of a swimming pool, you need endurance of your leg and arm muscles (the emphasis depending on which stroke you use). Once again, evaluating your upper and lower body separately will probably give you a more accurate assessment.

If your goal is to maintain your current degree of muscular endurance, then evaluating your success is easily achieved by taking note of which exercises you can perform and the number of repetitions you can achieve. Simply test yourself every month by repeating the same endurance challenge and assessing if you can still do it. After 12 weeks, an ability to perform the endurance exercises one level up (see Chapter Five) or to be able to perform twice the number of repetitions will demonstrate a substantial improvement in your endurance. If your goals exceed this, and you want to achieve levels of endurance greater than those in Level 4, then simply increase the repetitions. An ability to perform 25–30 repetitions of each exercise will demonstrate a good level of muscular endurance. Anything beyond that runs the risk of causing repetitive stress and invites boredom. Once you can perform 25–30 consecutive repetitions, you need to find a way to increase the intensity of the resistance. One way to do this is to slow down your execution of the movement. You may be surprised at how much harder the exercise is to perform when momentum is no longer assisting you.

Assessing the Endurance of Your Lower Body

How many times can you go up and down a staircase of at least 13 steps without pausing?

1. Three times? If not, most of the exercises in Level 1 of the lower body endurance programme will suit you to start with.

2. Six times? If not, most of the exercises in Level 2 of the lower body endurance programme will suit you to start with.
3. Nine times? If not, most of the exercises in Level 3 of the lower body endurance programme will suit you to start with.
4. Twelve times? If not, most of the exercises in Level 4 of the lower body endurance programme will suit you to start with.

If you can achieve this already, then work with Level 4 of the lower body endurance programme, but perform twice the number of repetitions.

Assessing the Endurance of Your Upper Body

How many times can you perform the following combination without pausing, while holding something that weighs 1 lb in each hand?
   a) Fully extend your arms out in front of you
   b) Keeping your upper arms parallel to the floor, bend your elbows and bring your hands back to your chest
   c) Fully extend your arms above your head
   d) Bring your hands back to your chest.

1. Five times? If not, most of the exercises in Level 1 of the upper body endurance programme will suit you to start with.
2. Ten times? If not, most of the exercises in Level 2 of the upper body endurance programme will suit you to start with.
3. Fifteen times? If not, most of the exercises in Level 3 of the upper body endurance programme will suit you to start with.
4. Twenty times? If not, most of the exercises in Level 4 of the upper body endurance programme will suit you to start with.

If you can already achieve this, then work with Level 4 of the upper body endurance programme, but perform twice the number of repetitions.

If pain in your joints is making you inflexible, your diet may be to blame.

Purines are found in all fish and meat products, especially poultry and beef. When purines are broken down by the liver, crystals of uric acid form and become deposited in the joints, resulting in irritation and inflammation.

Another cause of painful joints is the consumption of *antigens*, which are proteins foreign to the body. Once inside the body, antigens trigger the formation of antigen-antibody complexes by the body's immune system. This results in 'immune complex' diseases, including arthritis. Dairy products and eggs are exceptionally high in antigens and are the primary culprit in the formation of arthritis. In societies where animal products are seldom eaten arthritis is rare. For pain-free joints, increase your consumption of fresh raw fruits and vegetables.

Goal Setting and Measuring the Progress of Your Flexibility

Due to the age-related dehydration that gradually occurs as you get older, setting a goal simply to maintain your current degree of flexibility may be appropriate for you. This depends upon the range of movement you have at present. If you are supple enough to perform all the stretches in Level 4 of the flexibility programme, then your overall flexibility is sufficient for ease of movement, good posture, correct joint alignment and reduced injury risk. Anything less than that and you need to develop this aspect of your fitness. As a result of the law of specificity, the flexibility of your muscles may vary greatly. Once again, the occupations and lifestyles you have had will be influential factors. For example, if you have spent most of your working life sitting at a desk, it is likely that the muscles of the front of your chest (pectorals), back of your thighs (hamstrings) and front of your hips (hip flexors) will have restricted movement ranges. If your lifestyle includes a significant amount of swimming, then it is probable that the muscles of your shoulders have an above average degree of flexibility. The tests below will provide you with an indication of which level of the flexibility programme to begin with. It is especially relevant for this fitness component that you follow the instructions given in Chapter Five for creating your own *personalized* flexibility training programme.

If your goal is to maintain your current level of flexibility, ascertain which of the stretches in the programme take your muscles to the end of their ranges and perform them each day. If you work on developing your flexibility, being able to perform the stretch positions one level up from where you started after 12 weeks of practice will demonstrate a substantial improvement. If your flexibility goals exceed being able to achieve the stretches in Level 4, then pursuing yoga will provide you with a way to achieve those. There are numerous excellent books available on the subject, but investing in the services of a qualified yoga teacher, at least to begin with, would serve you well.

Assessing the Flexibility of Your Lower Body

1. Can you sit upright on the floor with your legs straddled and your knees straight? If not, most of the exercises in Level 1 of the lower body flexibility programme will probably suit you to start with.
2. Can you sit on the floor with your legs straddled and, keeping your knees straight, hold on to your knees? If not, most of the exercises in Level 2 of the lower body flexibility programme will probably suit you to start with.
3. Can you sit on the floor with your legs straddled and, keeping your knees straight, hold on to your calves? If not, most of the exercises in Level 3 of the lower body flexibility programme will probably suit you to start with.
4. Can you sit on the floor with your legs straddled and, keeping your knees straight, hold on to your feet? If not, most of the exercises in Level 4 of the lower body flexibility programme will probably suit you to start with.

If you can already achieve this, then follow Level 4 of the lower body flexibility training programme and strive to increase the range of movement within each position.

Assessing the Flexibility of Your Upper Body

1. Can you stand with your back and heels against a wall, and, keeping your arms straight, sweep them up overhead and touch the wall? If not, most of the exercises in Level 1 of the upper body flexibility programme will probably suit you to start with.
2. Can you perform this same movement (without leaning back) if you stand with your heels 3 in (7 cm) from the wall? If not, most of the exercises in Level 2 of the upper body flexibility programme will probably suit you to start with.
3. Can you perform this same movement (without leaning back) if you stand with your heels 8 in (20 cm) from the wall? If not, most of the exercises in Level 3 of the upper body flexibility programme will probably suit you to start with.
4. Can you perform this same movement (without leaning back) if you stand with your heels 12 in (30 cm) from the wall? If not, most of the exercises in Level 4 of the upper body flexibility programme will probably suit you to start with.

If you can already achieve this, then follow Level 4 of the upper body flexibility-training programme and strive to increase the range of movement within each position.

Goal Setting and Measuring the Progress of Your Motor Skills

The two aspects of your motor skills that have been included in the programme are balance and coordination. These two motor skills have significant influence on reducing your risk of falling, on improving your posture and on enhancing your physical grace. Motor skills respond as well to training as any other component of fitness. The goals that you set for yourself depend upon your current abilities and your reasons for wanting to develop these aspects of your fitness. If you can achieve all the challenges in Level 4 of the motor skills training programme, then you have a sufficient level of balance and coordination to practise good posture and minimize your risk of falling. Developing these skills beyond that may be necessary for your participation in certain sports, games or pastimes. This is the component of fitness where the law of specificity is most relevant of all. Just because you can coordinate and balance sufficiently to play hopscotch is no indication of whether or not you can dance! This delightfully fun aspect of fitness can be developed continually and in a diverse range of ways. Have fun and enjoy it!

Assessing Your Balance

When you try these tests, be sure to have something stable nearby, such as a wall or chair, to grab should you lose your balance.

1. Can you walk along a six-foot long line of string, placed along the floor, without stepping off it? If not, most of the exercises in Level 1 of the balance programme will probably suit you to start with.
2. Can you balance while standing on one leg for ten seconds? If not, most of the exercises in Level 2 of the balance programme will probably suit you to start with.
3. Can you balance while standing on one leg and swing your arms as if you were marching, for ten seconds? If not, most of the exercises in Level 3 of the balance programme will probably suit you to start with.
4. Can you balance while standing on one leg with your eyes closed for ten seconds? If not, most of the exercises in Level 4 of the balance programme will probably suit you to start with.

If you can already achieve Level 4 of the balance-training programme, then studying and practising advanced yoga or gymnastic-like positions that demand this skill will provide you with additional training.

Assessing Your Coordination

1. Can you pat the top of your head with one hand while rubbing your tummy in a circular motion with your other hand? If not, most of the exercises in Level 1 of the coordination programme will probably suit you to start with.
2. Can you march slowly on the spot while swinging your arms twice as fast as your legs are going? If not, most of the exercises in Level 2 of the coordination programme will probably suit you to start with.

3. Can you kick alternate legs out in front of you while reaching forward with the opposite arm at the same time? If not, most of the exercises in Level 3 of the coordination programme will probably suit you to start with.

4. Can you conduct three-time with one hand (as if drawing a triangle in the air) while you conduct four-time with the other (stroke down – across to the left – over to the right – then back up)? If not, most of the exercises in Level 4 of the coordination programme will probably suit you to start with.

If you can already achieve Level 4 of the coordination-training programme, then taking up a dance class of any type will provide you with a fun and creative way to develop this skill further.

Planning for Fitness

It is far more natural to participate in some physical movement every day than it is to remain sedentary four or five days in a row and then exert yourself intensely on the remaining two or three days. In addition, the greater variety of activities that you participate in throughout any given week the broader your fitness abilities will be and the less you are at risk of sustaining an injury. The term used to describe the incorporation of a wide range of approaches to fitness is cross-training.

A very important aspect of any fitness regimen you undertake is adequate rest. Without this, your body will be unable to rise to the challenge of overload that brings about a training effect. Research indicates that it is a lack of recovery time, rather than high intensity of exercise, that typically leads to injury. As you get older, you will need proportionately greater rest and recovery periods between training sessions to allow for slower bodily responses.

FIT is a fun and useful acronym for the three considerations that need to be taken into account when planning any fitness programme:

F – stands for frequency, the number of times per week that you train any given aspect of your fitness.

I – stands for intensity, the strenuousness of the exercise.

T – stands for time, the duration of your exercise session.

The FIT recommendations for each fitness component are as follows:

Cardio-respiratory (Aerobic) Fitness

Frequency: Six to seven days per week. Even if you are starting out at Level 1 of the programme, it is better to take some moderate exercise each day rather than remain sedentary some days and exhaust yourself on others.

Intensity: It is valuable when training your aerobic capacity to become familiar with what it feels like to be exerting yourself at specific intensities. Heart rate monitoring may or may not be something that interests you. If it does, there are plenty of qualified fitness professionals who have the equipment and knowledge to enable you to use it. For the purposes of this book, it is recommended that you evaluate the intensity of your aerobic exertion by practising the use of the scale of perceived exertion.

Time: If you are starting out on Level 1 of the programme, you may only be able to achieve 3 on the scale of exertion for ten minutes or less. The recommended long-term goal is to be able to sustain a state of 4–5 on the scale of exertion for 60 minutes at a time.

1 = No effort.	No increase in my breathing rate or body temperature. This is not challenging me at all.
2 = Slight effort.	A slight increase in my breathing and an awareness that I am mildly exerting myself.
3 = Effort.	A notable increase in my breathing rate and I'm starting to feel warmer. This feels like exercise.
4 = Challenging.	I am breathing deeper and faster, my body temperature is significantly warmer and this feels like work.
5 = Demanding.	I can feel my heart beating faster and my breathing is deep and strong. I am getting hot, I can feel my muscles working, and I am really exerting myself.
6 = Distressing.	I cannot catch my breath, and my heart is beating very fast. This is no fun. I cannot continue at this intensity.

The recommended intensity for aerobic training is either 4 or 5 on the above scale. If you are recovering from illness or injury, or are significantly debilitated, then 3 is more appropriate. Once you reach 6 on the scale, you are no longer training your aerobic fitness but your anaerobic abilities. This means that you will not be getting the same benefits to your heart, lungs and bloodstream as explained in Chapter Three. The fitter and more efficient your cardio-respiratory system, the harder you will be able to work and still experience only 4 or 5 on the above scale of exertion.

Muscular Strength

Frequency: In order for your muscles to respond to strength training, they have to bring about actual growth within their muscle fibres. If the same muscles are challenged with overload on consecutive days, it does not allow the muscles the necessary opportunity to grow in between times. Therefore, you can either do your strength training on alternate days, or you can work certain muscles one day and others the next. If you are going to take this latter approach, then it is a good idea to work the muscles of your upper body and lower body on alternate days. This is because many muscles assist neighbouring muscles in bringing about certain movements and therefore might not be resting when you think they are. Although there is a slight cross-over in the vicinity of your pelvis, no muscles of the lower body work directly to bring about movements in your upper body, or vice versa.

Intensity: The degree of resistance that your muscles have to overcome, when training their strength, needs to be such that you cannot perform more than a maximum of 6–10 consecutive repetitions of the movement. The following levels of resistance are recommended according to which level of the programme you are starting out with:

Level One – work with resistances that tire your muscles after no more than 9–10 repetitions

Level Two – work with resistances that tire your muscles after no more than 8–9 repetitions

Level Three – work with resistances that tire your muscles after no more than 7–8 repetitions

Level Four – work with resistances that tire your muscles after no more than 6–7 repetitions.

Time: An effective way to develop your strength is to work in sets of 4–6 repetitions. A 'set' is a number of repetitions performed consecutively followed by a rest period. The rest period needs to be at least as long as it took you to perform the set of repetitions. It is recommended that you start out with just one set at each level of the strength training programme, increasing it to 2, 3 and then 4 sets before moving on to the next level. Once you achieve Level 4, you can begin to work towards performing 6 sets of each exercise.

Muscular Endurance

Frequency: The changes that take place as a result of muscular endurance training are different from those brought about by challenging your strength. It is acceptable to train your endurance 6–7 days per week, if you choose to do so. Three to 5 days per week is, however, sufficient to bring about positive changes. If you are starting out after many years of being sedentary, twice per week may be enough for you to begin with.

Intensity: The degree of resistance that your muscles have to overcome when training their endurance needs to be such that you cannot perform more than a minimum of about 12–15 consecutive repetitions of the movement. The following levels of resistance are recommended according to which level of the programme you are starting out with:

Level 1 – work with resistances that tire your muscles after no more than 12–14 repetitions

Level 2 – work with resistances that tire your muscles after no more than 15–17 repetitions

Level 3 – work with resistances that tire your muscles after no more than 18–20 repetitions

Level 4 – work with resistances that tire your muscles after no more than 20–25 repetitions.

Time: 2 sets of repetitions are effective for training endurance. If you are starting out at Level 1, a single set of each exercise will probably be enough. Once you can achieve 2 sets of the allocated repetitions, move on to Level 2. For Levels 2, 3 and 4, strive to continue working in sets of two.

Flexibility

Frequency: Your muscles will actually become less flexible in just 24 hours of being sedentary. Performing stretches daily is therefore important if your ranges of movement are to be maintained.

Intensity: In order for your muscles to be stretched they need to be taken to the end of their current movement range. This requires body awareness on your part. Always ease into stretches very gently and only take them to the point where you feel the muscle being gently stretched. This will feel like a mild but pleasant tension. Under no circumstances force your body into extremes of movement that are beyond its present capability.

Time: If your goal is to maintain your current degree of flexibility, then holding your stretches, statically, for a minimum of 10 seconds will be sufficient. In order to increase your ranges of movement, you need to hold each stretch for at least 20 seconds. This is because once you have held it for 10 seconds the tension in the muscle will tend to relax more, enabling you to stretch it a little further. This may even occur a second time, resulting in you holding your stretch for a total of 30 seconds. This type of developmental stretching requires a high degree of body awareness and focus on how the muscle feels as you stretch. If you are starting out having been very sedentary for an extended period of time, or you are over 65 years old, it is recommended that you hold your stretches for only 4–6 seconds to begin with. This is because the connective tissue of your muscles may have a tendency to bond with itself, making it difficult for you to come out of the stretch. Once stretching feels comfortable, and you can move in and out of the stretches easily, then progress with the length of time you hold them for.

Motor Fitness (Balance and Coordination)

Frequency: There is no limit on how often you train your motor skills. Daily is ideal.

Intensity: The intensity simply needs to be sufficient to challenge you, but not so much as to shake your confidence or result in you falling.

Time: All activities that challenge motor skills demand concentration. As you progress, you can strive to maintain your focus for progressively longer durations. You may be able to pick up and follow a short pattern of dance steps, but could you remain coordinated for an entire dance?

Plateauing

There may come a time, during any aspect of your fitness training, when you seem to be making no progress. When this happens, it is best to change to a different exercise modality. For example, once your body has become used to brisk walking, there may be a slowing down in the development of your aerobic fitness. If this happens, the best thing to do is to challenge your body in a different way. For example, if you have been walking try cycling, or if you have been jogging try dancing. This applies even if you are striving for a high level of performance in one specific sport. The more varied your approaches to training any one of the fitness components, the less your risk of repetitive stress injuries and the greater your fitness versatility. You will probably enjoy your training more, too.

Preparing for Exercise

The armed forces use the following phrase – 'The Six Ps': Prior Proper Preparation Prevents Poor Performance. (Actually there is usually another P inserted before the word Poor, the slang for urinating, but we will not include it here!) The time and effort you invest in planning for your fitness regimen will pay massive dividends. Some aspects of preparation will simply enhance the effectiveness of your training, or increase your enjoyment of it. Other forms of preparation are vital to your health and safety.

The first thing to do is to ensure that you are physically healthy enough to train for the goals that you have set for yourself. It may be that seeking the advice of your health care professional is necessary. This is certainly true if you suffer from any of the following:

* Chest pain while at rest and/or during exertion
* A history of heart disease or stroke

- High blood pressure
- Diabetes
- Episodes of getting out of breath when you have only mildly exerted yourself or when you are resting
- Ulcerated wounds that don't seem to heal
- Unexplained weight loss, of ten pounds or more, over six months or less
- Pain in your legs when walking
- An irregular heartbeat when at rest
- Undergoing treatment for any heart, vascular, or lung problems
- Dizzy spells or episodes of fainting.

Even if you believe yourself to be healthy, asking your health-care professional to check you over before you begin is recommended.

Setting a Time

You are far more likely to adhere to your exercise programme if you develop the habit of doing it at a certain time of day. There is no fixed rule about when is best, except that it needs to be *before* a meal and not afterwards. Exercising while your body is trying to digest will result in poor performance of both activities. When you eat following exercise, you will actually digest, absorb, uptake, and assimilate the nutrients from your food far better than had you been sedentary before the meal.

Many people like to exercise first thing in the morning, and this does have various advantages. For one thing, the air is generally cleaner in the early morning than at any other time. Also life is full of surprises, and you never know what unexpected events might interfere with your schedule later in the day. Exercising in the evening may be the most realistic option for you, but it is not always ideal as the fatigue you accumulate during the day may dissolve your enthusiasm come the evening. The best and most natural option is to divide your exercise up into two or three sessions and do one session before each meal.

Once you have decided what time of day will generally suit you best to exercise, book it out in your diary as you would any other appointment to which you are committed. Make it known to family and friends that you will be unavailable during this time.

The degree to which they respect and honour your request will be a mirror of your own attitude towards your training.

Making the Space

If you plan on doing part or all of your exercise indoors, then you need to have the room to do it. Clearing furniture, tidying things away or moving other obstacles before each session will prove laborious and are likely to result in you abandoning the idea. Try at least to find a space where minimal preparation is needed in order for it to serve as your exercise area. Special attention needs to be paid to the floor surface of any exercise area. Rugs can be very dangerous as you can trip over them and fall. Even carpets can cause falls if you are moving on them wearing thick-soled exercise shoes, particularly if you are stepping sideways. Ensure any indoor exercise area you use is well ventilated. Of course, maximizing your time out of doors in fresh air and natural light is generally far preferable to being indoors. If you plan to start a hiking, walking, jogging, cycling or running programme, then a local ordinance survey map can be a great asset.

Equipment and Gear

Before you begin, be sure that you have obtained any necessary equipment and that it is all in good working order. Investing in the appropriate clothing is also important. This will enhance your safety as well as your enjoyment. It is best to dress in layers, as then you can remove or add clothing according to your body temperature. At the very least, you will need clothing that allows you to move freely, is not tight anywhere on your body (elastic waistbands are best) and is made of natural, breathable fibres. The right footwear depends almost entirely on the type of exercise that you choose. There is an enormous array of footwear available these days. There are shoes for every conceivable type of exercise and every sort of sport. Prices range from under £10 to several hundred. Generally with fitness and sports shoes, in terms of quality, you pay for what you get. To begin with, a good pair of what are referred to as cross-trainers will meet most of your needs and something in the range of £30 to £50 will serve you very well.

When buying fitness shoes, it is easy to get blinded by the technological sales pitch of the retailer. The best way to select a pair is simply by what feels comfortable to you. Avoid shoes that do not allow your foot to flex at the instep and be especially wary of buying any that are just that little bit too big, as they can lead to you tripping and falling while exercising. If you are exercising indoors and are not going to be either handling heavy equipment or jumping up in the air, then exercising with bare feet is not only acceptable, it is preferable. Feet are not naturally designed for shoes, and the more opportunities you get to allow them to move naturally without such restriction the better.

Finally, if you are a woman and plan on leaving the ground during your exercise sessions, such as in jogging, running, rebounding and many racket sports, then a supportive sports bra is a must.

Warming Up, Cooling Down

The older you get, the more important it becomes that you warm up properly before you exercise and cool down again afterwards. This is true regardless of the type of exercise you plan to undertake. The general aim of any warm-up is to allow your body to prepare itself for the more vigorous and demanding activities to follow. This involves redirecting blood from other places, such as your digestive tract, to the muscles that are going to be involved in the activity. Your body also needs to increase the speed at which your heart pumps, and increase the depth and rapidity of your breathing. It does these things in order to send a greater volume of blood and oxygen quickly around your body. The cartilage within your joints needs to be bathed in a greater quantity of synovial fluid, so that it can better protect your bone ends and act as effective shock absorbers.

The branch of your nervous system that transmits messages from your brain to your skeletal muscles needs to be 'tuned in'. The connective tissues within and around your muscles must become significantly warmer, enabling your muscle fibres and their inner structures to glide against each other easily, allowing your muscles to contract and stretch as necessary. Heat progressively generated from the preparatory movements of a warm-up also increases the pliability of your ligaments and the slight elasticity of your tendons. This means that both of these structures will be far less prone to being injured or damaged when stressed.

Performing a warm-up also allows you the time to switch to an awareness of your body on a physical level – listening to your body is absolutely vital to the safety and effectiveness of any exercise session.

Preparing Your Joints

Before exercising, you need to prepare each joint in turn by taking it a few times though its natural range of movement. This should be done slowly and without force. In order to do this, you need to know what ranges of movement each joint is designed to make. Your ankles are complex joints that provide a variety of movement possibilities. You can move your foot in a circle, point your toe down towards the floor, flex your foot so that your toes are higher than your heel and even turn your foot from side to side. Your knee joints are not as versatile. They are hinge joints and so are only designed to flex and extend. Any attempt at circling your knees can severely damage them. Your elbows are also hinge joints and therefore are designed for the same limited diversity of movements as your knees.

Your hip joints are put together totally differently from your elbows and knees. These are called ball and socket joints, which aptly describes their design. The top of each of your thighbones culminates in a ball-shaped mass of bone. This ball fits into the cup-shaped socket of your pelvis. You have the same arrangement at your shoulders. Ball and socket joints have the widest range of potential movements. This is why your legs and arms can move in almost any direction. The reason you can move your arms in a wider circle than you can your legs is because your hip sockets, for reasons of stability, are far deeper than those at your shoulders.

Your Spine

It is especially important that you understand the design and intended movement ranges of your spine if you are to take proper care of it. Your spine consists of 33 vertebrae, stacked up one on top of the other. The bottom four vertebrae, known as your coccyx, do not play any significant role in movement. Directly above your coccyx you have five vertebrae all fused together, which collectively form the back of your pelvis. These vertebrae are known as your sacrum, which joins with your pelvis at each of its outer edges at points known as your sacroiliac joints. These joints are what are known as semi-movable as opposed to freely movable. Although they do allow for a certain degree of pelvic movement, they can easily be damaged if twisted with force.

Where your spine ascends from your sacrum, you have another five segments known as your lumbar vertebrae. These are the largest vertebrae in your body, as they have to support the entire weight of your torso, head, and arms. Your lumbar vertebrae are designed to allow your torso to flex laterally. An example of lateral flexion is when you are sitting in a chair and lean over directly to the side to pick something up off the floor. Extending out from your lumbar vertebrae are finger-like projections of bone known as spinous processes. Any attempt to twist your lower back can result in these processes becoming jammed against each other. The ability for you to rotate your torso, such as you would do when you reach over into the back seat of the car while sitting in the front, is dependent upon your thoracic spine. This is the part of your spine that is directly above your lumbar spine, forming your upper back. It comprises of 12 vertebrae, all of which are designed for rotation of your torso. Unlike your lumbar spine, your thoracic area has very limited ability to accommodate lateral flexion. The uppermost part of your spine, situated at the back of your neck, comprises of the smallest of your vertebrae, because they only have to support the weight of your head. Here you have seven segments known as your cervical vertebrae. This area accommodates a wide range of movements. You can turn your head to the left and to the right, lift your chin up so that you can see the ceiling and drop it down so that you can see the floor. You can also tilt your head from side to the side.

Being encased within your spine protects your spinal cord. The circumference of your spinal cord is the same from top to bottom, whereas your vertebrae get progressively smaller the higher up your spine you go. The place where your spinal cord is most vulnerable is, therefore, at your neck. This is one of the reasons why movement of your neck should always be done with grace and awareness. Flinging your head backwards is a dangerous action, as it can impact upon this vital part of your central nervous system.

Now that you are a little more familiar with the design of your joints, you are in a position to mobilize them properly before undertaking strenuous exercise. By moving them several times slowly through their intended range of movements, you will stimulate the production of synovial fluid, increase the blood supply to your joints, and generate a warmth within the joints that will render the synovial fluid less viscous. The runnier the synovial fluid, the more your cushioning and shock absorbing cartilage will be able to absorb it, resulting in enhanced joint protection.

Preparing Your Muscles

Once you have prepared your joints, the next thing is to begin working your muscles so that a degree of warmth is generated from within them. This will also serve to initiate the necessary changes in your blood flow, heart rate and breathing rate. How you go about this depends upon the activity you are preparing for. If you are going out for a walk, begin at a meandering pace. If you are planning on jogging, start out walking. If running is your activity, then take a gentle jog to begin with.

For other types of activities, such as cycling and swimming, the same rule applies. Begin at a much lower intensity than you plan to achieve later. In order to generate heat in preparation for muscular strength or endurance training, perform the exact movements you intend to make but with very low resistance. For example, if you are training with free weights, start out with many repetitions of the movement before actually picking the weights up. If you are going to perform callisthenics, then adopt much easier positions to start with until you feel slightly warm.

Due to the extent of connective tissue within and around your muscles, it is vital that you do not attempt to train your flexibility until you have generated substantial warmth. The type of warmth needed for safe and effective stretching is that which is generated from within your muscles as a result of them working. Taking a hot bath or lying outside in the sun does not generate the same type of warmth and is therefore an inadequate preparation for flexibility training. The very best time to perform your stretches and develop your flexibility is directly after vigorous activity, such as aerobic or endurance training.

Cooling Down

This brings us on to the subject of cooling down after exercise. During physical exertion, blood is temporarily borrowed from other parts of your body in order to meet the needs of your working muscles. If you abruptly stop exercising, it places considerable strain upon your heart as it attempts to send the now excess volume of circulating blood back where it came from. Most types of exercise result in high volumes of blood being sent to your legs. Sudden discontinuation of activity can result in large quantities of blood gathering in your lower limbs, a situation that is compounded by the pull of gravity. When this blood pooling occurs, it also places great strain on the valves within your veins and can cause these blood vessels to become distorted and varicose. The way to cool down is simple; just perform your warm up in reverse. If you have been using your legs a lot, then make them the last thing you stop moving. You have a muscle in each of your calves called your soleus muscle which, when it contracts, presses against veins in the area and assists in returning blood back to your heart.

Once your breathing rate has returned to normal, but you are still feeling the warmth created by your earlier exertion, it is time to stretch out your muscles. This allows you to return your muscles to a longer and more relaxed state, aids in the recycling of lactates (which are naturally produced to some degree when you exert yourself physically), facilitates any necessary repair to your muscles and provides you with an opportunity to increase your flexibility.

Signs to Look Out For

The more experienced you become at exercising, the more you will be able to recognize when you are exerting too vigorously or too gently. Remember that the aim is to provide your body with a feasible challenge, not to stress it with unreasonable demands. Under-exerting is a problem, in as much as it is ineffectual. If you are just starting out after being sedentary for considerable time, the feelings that arise from physical exertion may be unfamiliar to you. If this is the case, you may under-exert out of anxiety. It is natural when you exercise that your breathing rate will quicken somewhat, your heart rate will increase and you will get warm. A reddening of your complexion is also quite natural. Some people go much redder than others, but this is not a sign that anything is wrong. Learning what the signs and symptoms are for heart attacks and strokes will help you to know the difference between your body's safe and natural responses to exercise and these life-threatening conditions.

Heart Attack and Stroke

A heart attack may cause crushing pains in your chest, upper back or left arm, accompanied by sudden dizziness, an ashen complexion, sweating and breathlessness. If you were having a heart attack, your pulse would be fast, irregular and weak, and your lips would turn blue. A stroke would cause you a sudden and severe headache and your pulse would be very strong. You would quickly become disorientated and probably sink into unconsciousness. The only three signs that can result from a healthful level of vigorous exercise, which can also be signs of either heart attack or stroke, are sweating, breathlessness and a faster *or* stronger pulse. As you can see, a heart attack would cause your pulse to be faster *and* weaker, and a stroke would cause it to become *stronger*. It is only vigorous exercise that will cause the heart to beat both faster *and* stronger. It is also especially useful to note that in the case of a heart attack your complexion would become paler, not redder as it can with exercise. I hope knowing this helps you to be less fearful of changes in your body as you exercise.

If you are *overdoing* it during your exercise session, any one or more of the following signs and symptoms may occur:

- A decline in coordination
- Pain in any given joint or muscle
- An inability to catch your breath
- Dizziness
- Weakness
- Nausea
- Trembling.

Overheating

As you get older, your body slowly becomes less efficient at cooling itself down when overheated. Diet and lifestyle factors that compound the problem include an unhealthy diet, consuming stimulants of any description and excess body fat. As an older exerciser, it becomes progressively important for you to be familiar with the symptoms of overheating, so that you can recognize early signals and take the necessary action to avert more serious problems. Heat exhaustion and heatstroke (commonly referred to collectively as sunstroke) are both conditions whereby your body has become depleted of water and mineral salts. Both occur because of intense action taken by the body in an attempt to cool itself down in the presence of extreme heat. Heat exhaustion is the milder form, while heatstroke is used to describe a severe physiological crisis. In its mildest form, loss of fluid and salts may result in symptoms of weakness, headache and nausea.

In severe cases, heatstroke can result in coma and even death. In cases where heat exhaustion or heatstroke has resulted from an overexposure to sunlight, it is not the light that has caused a problem, but the heat generated by the sun. The same conditions can result from subjecting the body to a sauna or undertaking intense physical training in hot environments. If at any time while exercising, especially in hot weather, you develop a headache and feel nauseous, then you need to take action.

The first thing to do is to find a way to cool your body down, such as removing layers of clothing and moving into a cooler environment. It is then vital that you replace the water and mineral salts that you have lost. The best way to do this is to drink water into which you have blended one or more bananas along with a few sticks of celery. If you do not have access to a blender, then drink water and eat bananas and celery at your earliest opportunity. The reason these foods help is because bananas are high in potassium and celery is high in sodium, both of which are needed for the rebalancing of your fluids on a cellular level. Under no circumstances should you eat table salt in an attempt to replace sodium, as it is actually an inseparable combination of sodium and chloride, and will result in severe further dehydration.

Most importantly, if you ever experience pain anywhere in your body, you should stop whatever it is that you are doing and investigate the cause. It may be something as simple as a blister caused by a rumple in your sock, but there is always the possibility that it is something more. Never work through pain of any description.

When Rest is Better than Play

Exercise is not the answer to everything, and sometimes it is inappropriate to be active.

Sickness

Whenever you feel unwell, in a way that is not your everyday experience, you need to rest your body rather then challenge it further with exercise. The old idea that you can 'burn off a cold' or 'exercise your way out of flu' is a dangerous misunderstanding of your body's needs and can result in life-threatening complications. Raising your body temperature, even if you have only a very slight fever, can end up causing you a serious health crisis. If your respiratory tract is congested or challenged in any way, the added burden of fitness training can result in permanent damage to your lungs. If you feel mildly ill-at-ease and are not sure if you are well enough or not to exercise, the best thing to do is to compromise and enjoy some gentle movement such as taking a slow walk in the fresh air and sunshine, or practising some non-strenuous yoga postures.

Injury

Injury is an obvious reason to stop exercising temporarily. Depending on your injury, it may be possible for you to continue training the uninjured parts of your body. For example, if you have hurt your ankle, this will not prevent you from sitting down and exercising your upper body. Similarly, if your shoulder is damaged, this is unlikely to prevent you from taking a walk.

Tiredness

Tiredness, beyond that caused by lethargy, is a sign not to exercise. A feeling of genuine tiredness is evidence that your body has insufficient energy at that time to conduct your basic metabolic processes. Placing further demands upon its already depleted state is therefore inappropriate. The cause of tiredness can be as simple as insufficient sleep, or it may be due to any number of dietary and/or lifestyle factors. If tiredness is a constant issue for you, then revisit Chapter One and make the necessary changes.

Over-training

It is possible that in your zeal you might have been over-training and that this is the cause of your feeling unwell. Should this occur, get plenty of extra rest, take a few days totally free of exercising, and use the time to reassess and restructure your fitness programme so that it is more realistic and health supporting. Signs that you have been over-training include insomnia, irritability, ever-present muscle aches or pains, pains in your joints, loss of appetite, a lack of motivation to exercise, reduced libido, headaches, an increase in your resting heart rate, a feeling that your legs are heavy and swollen lymph nodes.

Emotional Upsets

Traumas and the distressing events of life such as bereavement can be helped with physical activity. If you experience such difficult times, do what feels good to you whether it is rest or exertion. Be aware that being mentally distracted when you exercise can sometimes be dangerous. If you are going to use movement to help you overcome intensely distressing life episodes, do so with a mind to paying full attention to what you are doing.

Finally, if you have taken more than a week off from exercising, remember that you will have lost some degree of your fitness. Be sure to allow for this by expecting to perform with a little less intensity, and/or for a shorter duration, that you did before your break.

Now that you have made the necessary preparations, the time has come to get moving!

Chapter 5
Ready, Steady, Go!

If you have read the first four chapters, then you are ready to begin creating a fitter you! In this chapter you will find a wide range of safe and effective exercises to train your cardio-respiratory fitness, muscular strength, muscular endurance and flexibility. For each exercise there are four levels of ability for you to choose from. Level 1 exercises are the least physically demanding and Level 4 the most challenging. For each individual exercise start with Level 1, and then progress through each level until you find the one that slightly challenges you but feels attainable.

The programme is divided into four sections: cardiovascular, muscular strength, muscular endurance and flexibility. It is likely that you will be at a variety of different ability levels for exercises within one section. For example, within the muscular strength section you might be at Level 1 for the push-ups and Level 4 for lunges. The challenge is to have reached the next level, for each exercise, by the end of 12 weeks.

Before You Begin
Here is some general advice:

- ALWAYS prepare your body properly for exercise by warming up first (see Chapter Four)
- Regardless of the type of exercise you are doing, it will be both safer and more effective if you maintain correct posture as you perform it
- Never exercise to exhaustion
- Constantly listen to your body and understand that your ability level may vary from day to day
- Stop immediately if you experience any pain anywhere in your body other than what is, for you, a normal level of discomfort
- Ensure that you keep yourself well hydrated
- Dress in layers to avoid becoming cold or overheated

- If you are in any doubt about the suitability of any exercise for you, then consult your health-care professional.

Cardio-respiratory (Aerobic) Training

Points to Remember
When training your cardio-respiratory system it will serve you to become familiar with how it feels to be exerting at different intensities. Refer back to Chapter Four to familiarize yourself with the scale of perceived exertion. Always build up the intensity of work very gradually in any session and reduce it gradually at the end. Never exert yourself intensely, then suddenly stop and stand still. Doing so strains your heart, can cause varicose veins, and might cause you to feel dizzy or faint. Finally, avoid explosive movements as, being older, you will have some degree of increased connective tissue, making your ligaments and tendons somewhat more vulnerable to damage than those of a younger person.

Swimming, cycling, running and walking are all excellent for developing and maintaining aerobic fitness. There are, however, numerous other ways to challenge yourself aerobically (see Chapter Seven). Regardless of the approach you take, you can identify your starting point and evaluate your progress by testing your performance in any one of the following disciplines.

First, select your preferred form of exercise to test yourself with (swimming, cycling or running/walking), then begin with Level 1 and progress towards Level 4 until you find the level that challenges you but feels attainable. Your goal is then to develop your aerobic fitness, via any method you choose, until you can achieve the next level. This process can be repeated until you can achieve Level 4. If you discover that Level 4 is your starting point, then strive to progressively improve your time in 1-minute increments.

Swimming
To swim 400 metres (any stroke) in:

Level 1:	25 min
Level 2:	20 min
Level 3:	15 min
Level 4:	10 min

Cycling

To cycle 2 miles (on the flat) in:

Level 1:	25 min
Level 2:	20 min
Level 3:	15 min
Level 4:	10 min

Run/Walk

To travel 1 mile (on the flat) using nothing but your own legs in:

Level 1:	25 min
Level 2:	20 min
Level 3:	15 min
Level 4:	10 min

Muscular Strength, Endurance and Flexibility

Before undertaking the strength, endurance, or flexibility exercises below, please read the following important information.

Equipment

It is better for you to store your dumbbells and other heavy exercise equipment somewhere between hip and chest height, rather than on the floor. This will reduce the likelihood of you injuring your back when you go to pick them up. At the back of the book in Appendix 2 you will find listings of where you can obtain the necessary equipment.

Terminology

The term 'lock out' is used to describe when a joint is taken beyond simply being straight, into complete hyperextension. Locking out joints places them out of alignment, rendering them mechanically unstable and potentially damaging their surrounding structures.

In many of the exercises below you will be instructed to 'pull in your abdominals'. To do this, simply pull your belly button in towards your spine without rounding your back.

Reference is made to not allowing your bottom to 'stick out

behind you'. This has nothing to do with the size of your bottom but with the tilt of your pelvis. Weak abdominals and poor posture typically result in an exaggerated curve of the lower spine, potentially resulting in damage to that area and consequent pain. To prevent your bottom sticking out behind you, simply pull in your abdominal muscles and think of lifting your pubic bone upwards.

Transitions
Allow plenty of transition time between exercises to ensure you achieve good starting positions with correct technique and body alignment.

Balance
Avoid using a partner for balance, as you might both fall. If using a chair to help you to balance, place the chair against a wall to prevent it from sliding away from you should you suddenly lean on it heavily.

Effectiveness
In all exercises, strive for the widest ranges of pain-free movement. Every exercise can be slowed to a speed that feels comfortable to you and allows you to monitor your technique and movement ranges. It is far safer and much more effective to do fewer repetitions of a movement with good technique than it is to achieve a higher number with poor body alignment.

Strength-building Exercises
Remember, in order to build muscular strength, you need to perform exercises of an intensity that challenges you to perform six consecutive repetitions. When selecting your starting level for each of the exercises below, try the easiest first and then progress up through each level until you find the one that you can perform with correct technique but that challenges your strength by the sixth repetition. Do not progress to the next level until you can comfortably achieve four sets of six repetitions.

PUSH-UPS

Primary muscles exercised: The backs of upper arms (triceps), front of chest (pectorals), abdominals.

Level 1

Starting position: On your hands and knees, on a mat. Your knees should be about hip-distance apart and directly below your hips. Your hands should be shoulder-width apart and below your shoulders or slightly wider, with your hands facing forwards.

Movement: Keeping your feet and knees on the floor, slowly bend your elbows, lowering your face towards the floor. Then, using both arms, push yourself back up to the starting position.

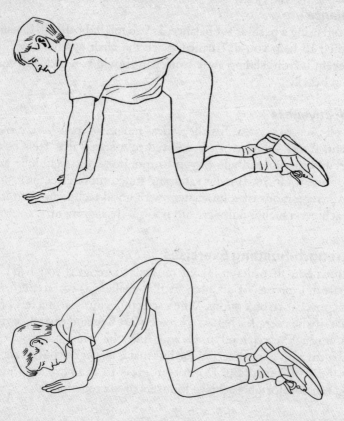

Push-ups Level 1

Essential technique:

• Throughout the exercise, ensure that your abdominal muscles are pulled in, holding your back flat like a table-top
• Keep your weight forward over your arms throughout the exercise
• Do not lock out your elbows on the way up.

Breathing: Inhale as you go down; exhale as you come back up.

Level 1 Alternative
If you are uncomfortable kneeling, or have difficulty in getting down onto the floor, wall push-ups provide an excellent alternative.

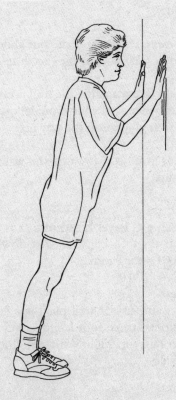

Push-ups Level 1 alternative

Starting position: Stand facing a wall with your feet hip-distance apart and facing forwards. You should be close enough to the wall that if you stand upright, with both arms extended straight out in front of you and with your fingers outstretched, you can just touch the wall.

Movement: Stand upright, with your abdominals held in tight, extend both arms out in front of you at shoulder height with your palms facing the wall. Keeping your back straight and your feet flat on the floor, allow your whole body to fall forwards from your ankles. Catch yourself with your hands against the wall before your face reaches it, allowing your elbows to bend as you do so. Keeping your abdominals pulled in and your back straight, use the strength in your arms to push yourself back to the starting position.

Essential technique:

- Throughout the exercise, ensure that your abdominal muscles are pulled in. Do not allow your hips to drop forward at any time
- Ensure your hand placing against the wall is correct; shoulder height and slightly wider than your shoulders
- Do not lock out your elbows on the way up.

Breathing: Inhale as you drop towards the wall; exhale as you push yourself back up.

Level 2

The exercise is the same as Level 1, except that as you lower your face to the floor you aim to bring your nose down about 6–8 in (15–20 cm) in front of your hands.

Level 2 Alternative

This exercise is the same as for wall push-ups (see above), but with your feet positioned three foot-lengths away from the wall. Allow your heels to raise up slightly off the floor as you drop forwards onto the wall.

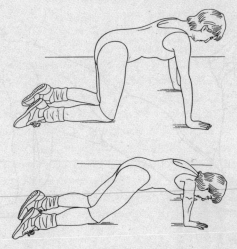

Push-ups Level 2

Level 3
Starting position: Lie face-down on a mat. Bend at the knees, lifting your lower legs up off the floor, and cross your ankles. Then slide your knees outwards until they are hip-distance apart. Place your hands on the floor at shoulder level, but slightly wider apart than your shoulders. Your hands should be facing forwards.
Movement: Keep your abdominals pulled in tight, so that your back does not sag. Then use the strength in your arms to lift your whole body, down as far as your knees, up from the floor. There should be a straight line from your shoulders to your knees throughout the exercise, and at no time should your bottom be stuck up in the air.
Essential technique:

- Aim to lift your shoulders and hips off the floor simultaneously (do not let the shoulders come up before the hips)
- Throughout the exercise, ensure that your abdominal muscles are pulled in, holding your back flat like a board
- Do not lock out your elbows on the way up

Breathing: Exhale as you push up; inhale as you lower yourself back down to the floor.

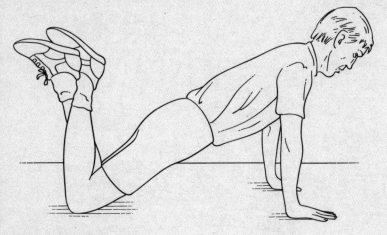

Push-ups Level 3

Level 3 Alternative

This exercise is the same as for Level 2 – extended wall push-ups (see above), but with your feet placed four foot-lengths away from the wall. Be especially careful to keep your abdominals pulled in tight so as not to let your hips fall forwards and your back arch as you drop onto the wall.

Level 4

Starting position: Lie face down on the floor. Place your hands, facing forwards, on either side of your shoulders. Tuck your toes under so that the pads of your toes are against the floor.

Movement: Pulling your abdominals in very tightly, and keeping your back straight, use the strength in your arms to lift your chest, hips, and legs up off the floor as one piece. Continue until your arms are fully extended, but do not lock out your elbows. Lower yourself back down, under control, returning to the starting position.

Essential technique:

- Be sure to lift your body and legs as one unit; do not lift your chest in advance of lifting your hips
- Throughout the exercise, ensure that you maintain one continual straight line from your shoulders to your ankles

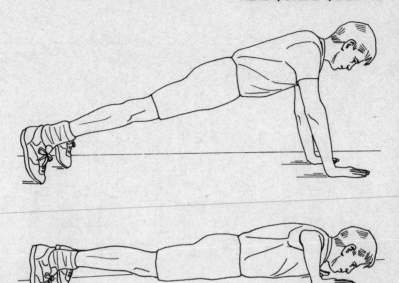

Push-ups Level 4

• Keep your abdominals pulled in very tightly so as not to let your belly drop towards the floor and your back arch
• At no point should your bottom be stuck up in the air
• Do not lock out your elbows on the way up; keep them soft.

Breathing: Inhale as you go down; exhale as you come back up.

SIT AND STAND
Primary muscles exercised: Fronts of thighs (quadriceps), buttocks (gluteus maximums), and backs of thighs (hamstrings).

Level 1
Starting position: Sit upright, towards the edge of a chair, with your feet placed hip-distance apart and flat on the ground with a right angle at your knees. Your hands should be resting on your thighs.
Movement: Leading with your shoulders, but using the strength

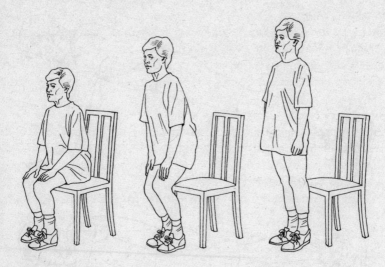

Sit and Stand

in your legs, push yourself to a standing position. Then, lowering yourself under control, return to the starting position.
Essential technique:

- Do not let your knees roll inwards as you stand; keep them in alignment with your ankles throughout the movement.

Breathing: Exhale as you stand and inhale as you lower yourself back to a sitting position.

Level 2
The same as Level 1, but with your hands clasped behind your back.

Level 3
The same as Level 1, but holding a 5 lb weight in your hands a few inches in front of your abdominals.

Level 4
The same as Level 1, but holding an 8 lb weight in your hands a few inches in front of your abdominals.

INCLINED PLANE

Primary muscles exercised: Buttocks (gluteus maximus), back (erector spinae), backs of thighs (hamstrings), backs of shoulders (posterior deltoids), upper back (trapezius and rhomboids), backs of upper arms (triceps).

Level 1

Starting position: Sit on the floor with your legs together and straight out in front of you. Lean back slightly from the hips and place your hands flat on the floor, facing forwards and shoulder width apart. Straighten your arms.

NB: You may find it more comfortable for your wrists if you place a rolled-up mat under your hands.

Movement: Keeping your knees straight, and pointing your toes away from you, use the muscles of your buttocks and back to lift your hips towards the ceiling until you feel your bottom just lose contact with the floor. Lower your hips back down again.

Essential technique:

- Keep your abdominal muscles pulled in tight to support your back
- Do not lock out your elbows

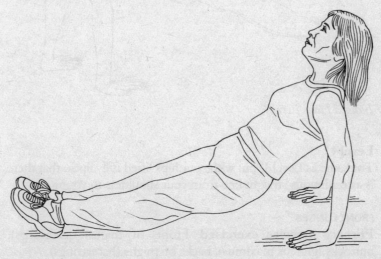

Inclined Plane Level 1

- Keep your neck long and look up towards the ceiling as you lift your hips.

Breathing: Exhale as you lift your hips and inhale as you return to the starting position.

Level 2
The same as Level 1, but lifting your bottom well clear of the floor this time.

Level 3
The same as Level 1, but with your hips lifted high enough so that your toes are touching the floor.

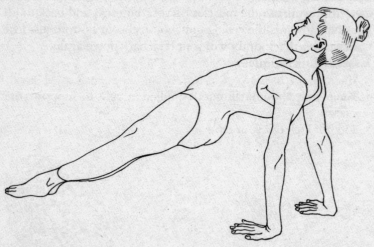

Inclined Plane Level 4

Level 4
The same as Level 1, but with your hips lifted fully up so that there is a continuous straight line from your shoulders to your toes.

FRONT LUNGES
Primary muscles exercised: Fronts of thighs (quadriceps), buttocks (gluteus maximus), backs of thighs (hamstrings).

Level 1

Starting position: Stand sideways next to a chair back with it slightly in front of you. Reach forward and hold on to the chair back with the hand nearest to it. Place your feet hip-distance apart and facing forwards. With the leg that is furthest away from the chair, take a large step forwards (large enough so that the heel of your other foot has to rise up off the floor). Keep your abdominals pulled in and your back straight.

Movement: Bend both knees, allowing your back heel to rise up off the floor as necessary, until the knee of your back leg is about 6 in (15 cm) from the floor. Using the strength in your legs, push yourself back up to the starting position.

This exercise needs to be done on both sides (with both the right and left leg in front).

Essential technique:

- Keep your back upright throughout the exercise; do not tip forwards from the hips
- Maintain the position of your feet hip-width apart at all times
- Look straight ahead throughout the movement

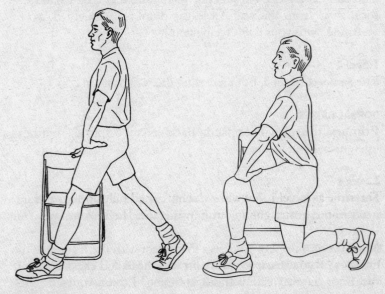

Front Lunges

- Ensure that your front knee remains over your ankle joint and does not jut out in front of your toes
- Keep your weight evenly distributed over both legs. As you bend, think of lowering the centre of your crotch straight down towards the floor
- If you need to, use your arm strength on the chair to help you get back up.

Breathing: Inhale as you bend your knees and exhale as you push yourself back up.

Level 2
The same exercise as Level 1, but bend until the knee of your back leg is just short of touching the floor. You may need to build up to this gradually. Also, do this standing next to a wall instead of using a chair. This will still help you to balance, but will no longer provide you with a way to use your arms to get back up.

Level 3
The same as Level 2 but holding a 5 lb dumbbell in the hand furthest away from the wall. Hold the dumbbell straight down by your side, with your palm facing you.

Level 4
The same as Level 3, but increasing the weight to an 8 lb.

DORSAL RAISES
Primary muscles exercised: Back (erector spinae), buttocks (gluteus maximus).

Level 1
Starting position: Lie, face down, on a mat, with your forehead to the ground and your hands resting behind you on your bottom.
Movement: Keeping your feet in contact with the floor, use the muscles of your back to slowly lift your head and chest as far off the floor as you can without straining. Lower yourself back down, under control.

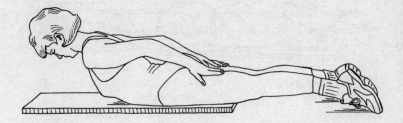

Dorsal Raise Level 1

Essential technique:

- Look down towards the floor throughout the exercise
- If you feel any discomfort in your lower back, do not rise up so far
- Do not allow your feet to lose contact with the floor at any time.

Breathing: Exhale as you lift up; inhale as you lower back down.

NB: If you have severe kyphosis (exaggerated curvature of the upper back), this exercise is not suitable for you. The following is an alternative:

Starting position: Stand with your back to a wall and your heels against the bottom of it.

Movement: As you inhale, stand up as straight as you can and lengthen your neck. Then press your shoulders, and the back of your head, back towards the wall. Exhale and release.

Breathing: Exhale as you lift up; inhale as you lower back down.

Level 2

The same exercise as Level 1, but with your arms in the following position:

Lying face down, with your forehead to the floor, extend both arms straight out along the floor at shoulder height. Bend your elbows to a right angle, with your palms facing the floor. Use the muscles of your back to lift your head and chest up off the floor, while simultaneously lifting your arms. Lower your body back down under control.

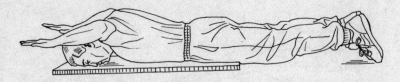

Dorsal Raise Level 2

Level 3
The same exercise as Level 1, but with your arms extended straight out along the floor above your head. Use the muscles of your back to lift your head and chest up off the floor, while simultaneously lifting your arms. Keep your upper arms close to your ears throughout the movement. Lower your body back down under control.

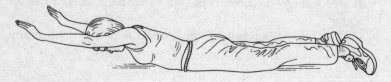

Dorsal Raise Level 3

Level 4
The same as Level 3, but holding an object, such as a large book weighing about 3 lb, between your hands. Remember not to let your feet lift from the floor.

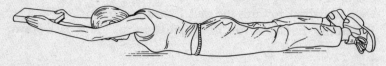

Dorsal Raise Level 4

BICEPS CURLS
Primary muscles exercised: Front of upper arms (biceps).

Level 1

Starting position: Stand upright with your feet hip-distance apart. Ensure your bottom is not stuck out behind you. Hold a 5 lb weight down in front of you between your hands, with your palms facing forwards. Have your elbows almost straight, but not locked. Pull in your abdominals.

Movement: Keeping your elbows close to the sides of your body, bring the weight up towards your chest by bending your elbows. Lower the weight back down under control.

Essential technique:

- Do not lean back from the hips as you lift the weight
- Maintain a good upright stance throughout and look straight ahead.

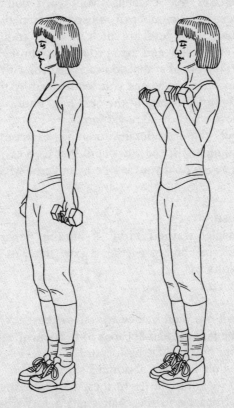

Biceps Curls

Breathing: Exhale as you lift the weight, inhale as you lower it back down.

Level 2

The same as Level 1, but holding an 8 lb weight.

Level 3

The same as Level 1, but holding a 5 lb weight in each hand.

Level 4

The same as Level 1, but holding an 8 lb weight in each hand.

Exercises for Endurance Development

In order to develop greater muscular endurance, you need to perform exercises that challenge you when you attempt to perform an extended number of consecutive repetitions. When selecting your starting level for each of these endurance exercises, try the easiest first and then progress up through each level until you find the one that that you can perform with the correct technique, but that challenges your endurance by the fifteenth repetition. Do not progress to the next level until you can comfortably achieve 2 sets of 20 repetitions.

Throughout these endurance-training exercises, maintain regular breathing at a speed and depth that feels comfortable to you. Be sure not to hold your breath at any time while performing them.

FRONT LEG RAISE

Primary muscles trained: Front of hip (hip flexors), front of thighs (quadriceps), and to a lesser degree, inner thighs (adductors) and abdominals.

Level 1

Starting position: Stand sideways on to the back of a chair. Hold the chair with the hand nearest to it. Stand up tall with your feet under your hips and facing forward.

Movement: Pull in your abdominals to support your back. Transfer your weight to the leg furthest away from the chair, then slide the foot nearest to the chair straight forwards along the floor in front of you, without placing any weight on it. Keep your supporting leg straight, but not locked out at the knee. Once the foot is as far in front of you as it can go without affecting the rest of your posture, lift the whole leg from the hip until the foot is about 6–12 in (15–20 cm) off the floor. Lower the leg back down and return to the starting position.

Essential technique:

- Do not sink down into the supporting hip; think of lifting your weight up and out of your hips as you work
- Do not swing the leg, but be deliberate and controlled in your movements
- Maintain an upright stance throughout the exercise; do not lean back from the hips as you lift the leg.

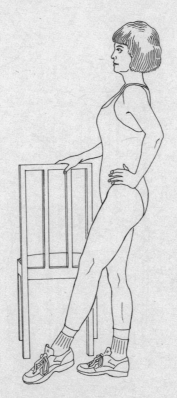

Front Leg Raise Level 1

Level 2

The same exercise as Level 1, but lifting your foot 12–18 in (20–25 cm) off the floor.

Level 3

The same exercise as Level 2, but wearing a 2 lb ankle weight.

Level 4

The same exercise as Level 3, but wearing a 3 lb ankle weight.

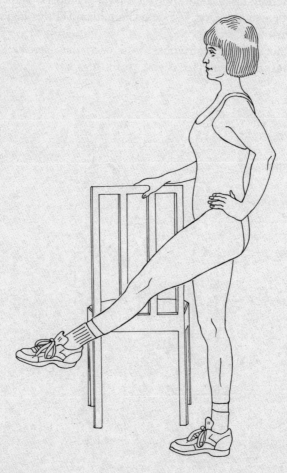

Front Leg Raise Level 2

FRONT ARM RAISE

Primary muscles trained: Front of shoulders (anterior deltoids) and top of shoulders (medial deltoid).

Level 1

Starting position: Stand upright with your feet hip-distance apart. Pull in your abdominals. Let your arms hang down by your sides, making soft fists with your hands. Turn the backs of your fists to face forwards. Relax your shoulders back and down.

Movement: Slowly raise your arms straight up in front of you until your fists are level with your shoulders. The backs of your fists should be facing the ceiling. Lower both arms under control back to the starting position.

Essential technique:

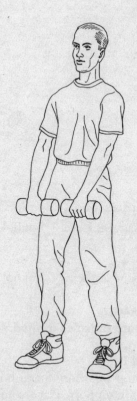

- Keep your abdominals pulled in throughout the movement and do not let your bottom stick out behind you
- Your elbows should be straight but not locked
- Remain upright in your posture; do not lean back as you lift your arms.

Level 2

The same as Level 1, but holding a 3 lb dumbbell in each hand.

Front Arm Raise

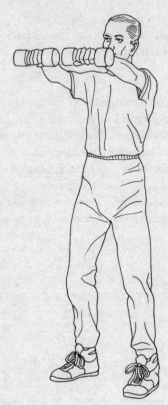

Front Arm Raise

Level 3
The same as Level 1, but holding a 5 lb dumbbell in each hand.

Level 4
The same as Level 1, but holding an 8 lb dumbbell in each hand.

CALF RAISES
Primary muscles trained: Calves (gastrocnemius and soleus).

Level 1
Starting position: Stand holding onto the back of a chair or a wall for support. Place your feet hip-distance apart and facing forward.

Movement: Rise up a little way onto the balls of your feet so that your heels just come off the floor. Lower back down under control.

Essential technique:

- Ensure that you centre your weight over your big toes and do not roll out over your little toes
- Pull up through the fronts of your thighs as you perform the movement but do not lock out your knees
- Do not let your bottom stick out behind you.

Level 2
The same as Level 1, but lifting right up, as high as you can, onto the balls of the feet.

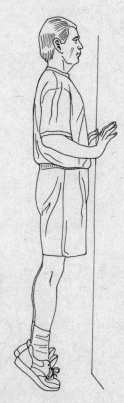

Calf Raises Levels 1 and 2

Level 3

Starting position: Stand on a step (a staircase works well). Holding onto the wall or banister for balance, place the balls of your feet on the edge of the step and allow your heels to drop down below the level of your toes. Pull in your abdominals and stand with your knees straight but not locked.

Movement: Rise all the way up onto the balls of your feet, then lower your heels back down back again below the level of your toes.

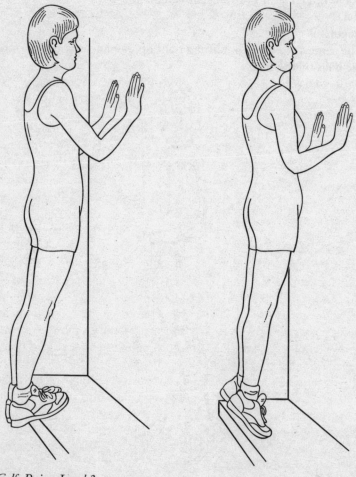

Calf Raises Level 3

Essential technique:

• Ensure that you centre your weight over your big toes and do not roll out over your little toes
• Pull up through the fronts of your thighs as you perform the movement but do not lock out your knees
• Do not let your bottom stick out behind you
• Execute the movement in a controlled manner.

Level 4
The same as Level 3, but with the addition of wearing 2 lb ankle weights.

OVERHEAD PRESS
Primary muscles trained: Tops of shoulders (medial deltoids), backs of upper arms (triceps), top of back (trapezius), sides of neck (sternocleidomastoid).

Level 1
It is important that you learn how to get into the starting position for this exercise correctly at Level 1. Otherwise, when you attempt to perform the exercise with dumbbells in Levels 2, 3, and 4, you might injure yourself.
Starting position: Stand upright with your feet hip-distance apart and your abdominals pulled in. With your arms relaxed down by your sides, make your hands into soft fists with your palms facing your thighs. Lift both arms up and out to the side until they reach shoulder height (the backs of your fists should be facing upwards). Next, turn your arms so that your thumbs are uppermost. Then, keeping your upper arms still, flex at the elbows until your knuckles are pointing straight to the ceiling. You are now ready to begin.
Movement: Looking straight ahead, push your fists up towards the ceiling until your elbows are straight but not locked. Lower your elbows back down until they are again level with your shoulders. To come out of the exercise lower the elbows to shoulder height, and then straighten them before slowly bringing both arms back down by your sides.

NB: Perform this exercise from a chair if you have a lower back problems.

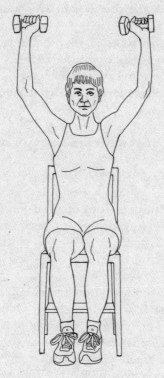

Overhead Press

Essential technique:

* Look straight ahead throughout the exercise
* Avoid hunching your shoulders as you extend your arms upwards
* Keep your abdominals pulled in throughout and do not let your bottom stick out behind you
* Between each repetition, only lower your elbows to shoulder height, no lower.

Level 2
The same as Level 1, but holding a 3 lb dumbbell in each hand.

Level 3
The same as Level 1, but holding a 5 lb dumbbell in each hand.

Level 4
The same as Level 1, but holding an 8 lb dumbbell in each hand.

HAMSTRING CURLS
Primary muscles trained: Back of thighs (hamstrings).

Level 1
Starting position: Lie face down on the floor with your forehead resting on the backs of your hands.
Movement: Keeping your thighs side by side on the floor, bring your right heel as close towards your right buttock as you can, then lower it back down to the floor. When you have performed the appropriate number of repetitions, repeat with the left leg.

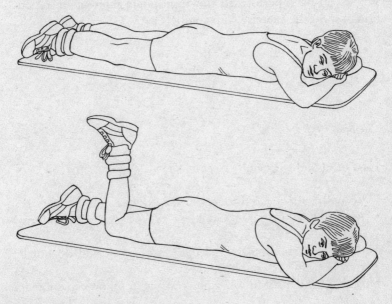

Hamstring Curls Level 1

NB: If you feel any discomfort in your lower back, place a pillow under your hips.

Essential technique:

* Do not fling the leg to and fro, but rather move it in a controlled and deliberate way.

Level 2

Starting position: Hold on to the back of a chair. Take one step back from the chair and incline slightly forwards from the hips. Place your feet hip-distance apart and facing forwards. Lift up from your pelvis and pull in your abdominals. Extend your right foot back behind you on the floor as far as it will go, keeping your supporting leg straight.

Movement: Without moving your right thigh, bring your right heel up as close to your right buttock as you can by bending your knee, and then lower it back down to the floor under control. When you have performed the appropriate number of repetitions, repeat the exercise with your left leg.

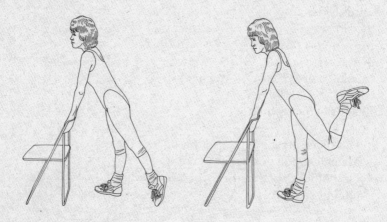

Hamstring Curls Level 2

NB: If you suffer from arthritis in your hips or knees, perform the exercise alternately with each leg until your have achieved your goal number of repetitions on both sides.

Essential technique:

- Do not fling the working leg to and fro, but rather move it in a controlled and deliberate way
- Do not lock out the knee of your supporting leg.

Level 3
The same as Level 2, but wearing a 2 lb ankle weight.

Level 4
The same as Level 2, but wearing a 5 lb ankle weight.

LATERAL ARM RAISE
Primary muscles trained: Top of shoulders (medial deltoid).

Level 1
Starting position: Stand upright, with your feet hip-distance apart, and abdominals pulled in. Relax your arms straight down in front of you, and form soft fists with your hands. Place your knuckles together and have the back of your hands facing outwards. Your arms should be almost straight with a slight bend at the elbows.
Movement: Lift both of your arms up and out to the sides until they reach shoulder height, whereby the backs of your hands should be uppermost. Lower back to the starting position under control.
Essential technique:

- Look straight ahead of you throughout the exercise
- Maintain good posture at all times
- Do not lean backwards as you lift your arms; maintain a solid upright stance.

Level 2
The same as Level 1, but holding a 3 lb dumbbell in each hand.

Level 3
The same as Level 1, but holding a 5 lb dumbbell in each hand.

Level 4
The same as Level 1, but holding an 8 lb dumbbell in each hand.

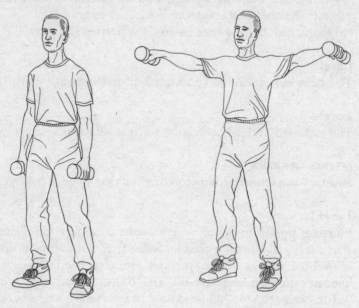

Lateral Arm Raise

LATERAL LEG RAISE
Primary muscles trained: Outsides of thighs (abductors).

Level 1
Starting position: Lie on your right side on a mat using your arm, or a pillow, to support your head in a way that is comfortable for you. Lie with your body straight (not flexed at the knees or hips), with your left leg resting directly on your right leg. Place the palm of your left hand on the floor in front of your body to prevent yourself from rolling forwards. Keeping your knees together, and without moving your thighs, slide your lower legs back behind you by bending at the knees. There should be a straight line from your chest to your knees. Pull in your abdominals.

Movement: Keeping your left knee bent, lift your entire left leg up towards the ceiling, keeping the outside of your thigh uppermost. Then lower your leg back down under control. Once you have completed the appropriate number of repetitions, lie on your left side and repeat the exercise with your right leg.
Essential technique:

• Keep your abdominals pulled in throughout the exercise.

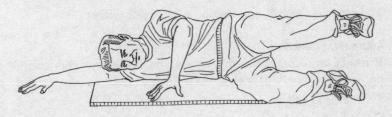

Lateral Leg Raise Level 1

Level 2
Starting position: Similar to Level 1, but this time, keeping your left leg straight.
Movement: Keeping your left leg straight, with your toes pointed slightly downwards towards the floor, lift your leg as high as you can directly towards the ceiling. Lower your leg back down under control.
Essential technique:

• Keep your abdominals pulled in throughout the exercise

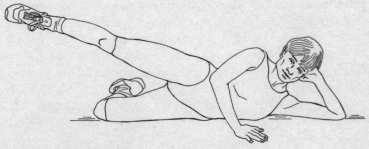

Lateral Leg Raise Level 2

- As you lift your left leg, keep your toes pointing slightly down towards the floor, and your left knee facing forwards. Do not allow your hip to drop back or your knee to face the ceiling
- Lower under control; do not let the leg drop back down.

Level 3
The same as Level 2, but wearing a 2 lb ankle weight.

Level 4
The same as Level 2, but wearing a 5 lb ankle weight.

ABDOMINAL CURLS
Primary muscles trained: The abdominals (rectus abdominis, transverse abdominis), pelvic floor (including illiococcygeus and pubococcygeus).

Level 1
Starting position: Lie on your back on the floor, with your knees bent up and both feet flat on the floor hip-distance apart. Allow a natural curve to be present in your lower back.
Movement: Contract your pelvic floor by pulling up the muscles inside your crotch (the same muscles that you use to retain urine and/or faeces when you need to go to the toilet and are unable to). Pull your belly button in towards your spine. Keeping your buttocks on the floor, roll your lower back into the mat while tilting your pubic bone towards your belly button. Release, and return to the starting position, relaxing your abdominals and pelvic floor.

   NB: See Chapter Three for more information about your pelvic floor.

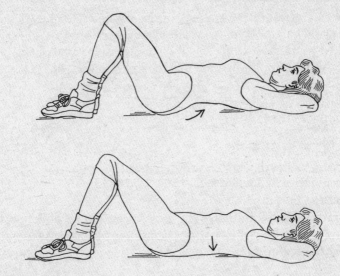

Abdominal Curls Level 1

Essential technique:

• Keep your feet in light contact with the floor; resist pushing down hard with them as you perform the exercise

• Maintain comfortable breathing throughout. Do not hold your breath.

Level 2

Starting position: Lie on your back on the floor, with your knees bent up and both feet flat on the floor hip-distance apart. Allow a natural curve to be present in your lower back. Place the palm of one hand low down on the back of your head (not on your neck). Place the other hand on the top of the thigh nearest to it.

Movement: Pull up your pelvic floor muscles and pull your belly button towards your spine. Keeping your chin a hand-width away from your chest, and looking towards the top of the wall in front of you, lift your head and shoulders up off the floor. Come up only as high as your abdominal muscles can lift you; do not strain and *do not attempt to sit all the way up*. Lower yourself back down under control, and then relax your abdominals and pelvic floor.

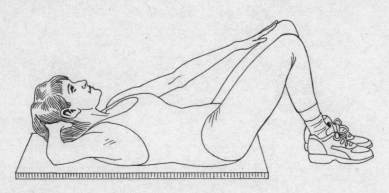

Abdominal Curls Level 2

Essential technique:

- Keep your chin a hands-width away from your chest through-out the exercise
- Your hand is to offer support to your head only; do not pull on your head
- Keep your feet on the floor throughout the exercise; do not let them lift
- The back of your pelvis (sacrum) should not lose contact with the floor at any time during the exercise
- Exhale as you curl up and inhale as you lower yourself back down.

Level 3
The same as Level 2, but with both hands on the back of your head with the elbows pressed back. Remember – do not pull on your head and keep your chin well away from your chest through-out the movement.

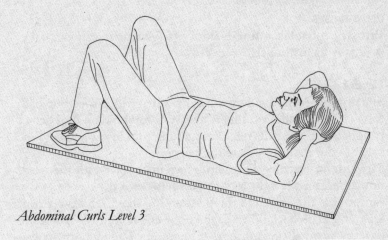

Abdominal Curls Level 3

Level 4

The same as Level 2, but with both arms stretched out straight above your head. Keep your upper arms next to your ears throughout the movement. Do *not* swing your arms forward to assist you with the exercise.

NB: If your neck is not strong enough to keep your head from dropping backwards as you curl up, then be sure to use one hand to support it. You can still extend the other arm above your head, and you can hold a light weight in that hand if you need added resistance for your abdominals.

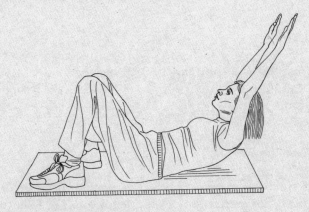

Abdominal Curls Level 4

GLUTE RAISES

Primary muscles trained: Buttocks (gluteus maximus), backs of thighs (hamstrings).

Level 1

Starting position: Lie face down on a mat with a rolled up bath towel, or mat, under your hips. Rest your forehead on the back of your hands. Bend your right knee, lifting your lower leg, until the sole of your right foot faces the ceiling.

Movement: Keeping both hip bones in contact with the towel or mat, push your right foot as far up towards the ceiling as you can, so that the knee and thigh lift up off the floor. Lower your knee and thigh back down to the floor under control. When you have performed the appropriate number of repetitions, repeat the exercise using your left leg.

NB: If you experience any discomfort in your lower back, use a larger roll under your hips.

Essential technique:

- Execute the movement smoothly; do not kick with the leg
- Only lift the leg as high as it will go without lifting the hip up off the floor.

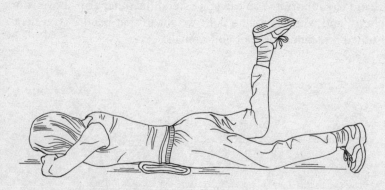

Glute Raises Level 1

NB: If you have severe kyphosis (exaggerated curvature of the upper back) this exercise is not suitable for you. The following is an alternative:

Starting position: Lean with your forearms resting on a waist-high surface (such as a table). Place your feet hip-distance apart and facing forwards.

Movement: Extend one foot out along the floor behind you, keeping your leg straight. Pull in your abdominals and then, keeping both hips facing forwards, lift the leg up behind you as far as you can without swinging out at the hip. Lower it back down under control. If you experience any discomfort in your back, you are attempting to lift the leg too high.

Essential technique:

- Your hips should both face forwards throughout the exercise
- Keep the back of the knee uppermost as you lift the leg
- Aim to execute the movement smoothly; do not kick the leg up.

Level 2
The same as Level 1, but without bending at the knee. Keep the leg you are lifting straight, throughout the exercise, with the toe pointed away from you.

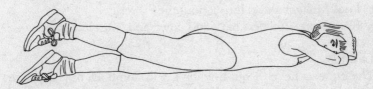

Glute Raises Level 2

Level 3
The same as Level 2, but wearing a 2 lb ankle weight.

Level 4
The same as Level 2, but wearing a 4 lb ankle weight.

LATERAL INCLINES
Primary muscles trained: The abdominals (internal obliques, and transverse abdominis), and the lower back (quadratus lumborum).

Level 1

Starting position: Sit towards the edge of a chair, with your feet slightly wider apart than the chair legs. The chair needs to be of a height that places you with a right angle at your knees. Allow your arms to hang naturally down by your sides. Sit upright, lifting up out of your hips, with your abdominals pulled in.

Movement: Keeping your right shoulder back so as to prevent you from tipping forwards, lean directly over to the right as far as you can go without your left buttock losing contact with the chair. Return to the starting position. When you have performed the appropriate number of repetitions, repeat the exercise leaning to the left.

Essential technique:

- Both buttocks should remain in contact with the chair throughout the exercise
- Lean directly to the side; do not tip forwards or backwards
- Ensure that your knees remain in alignment over your ankles and do not roll in as you lean over
- Only lean as far as you are able to without tipping forwards; do not attempt to touch the floor
- Look straight ahead throughout the exercise
- Keep your shoulders back and down and your neck long.

Level 2

The same as Level 1, but holding a 3 lb dumbbell in the *opposite* hand from the side you are leaning.

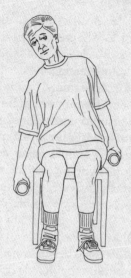

Lateral Inclines

Level 3
The same exercise as Level 1, but holding a 5 lb dumbbell in the *opposite* hand from the side you are leaning.

Level 4
The same as Level 1, but holding an 8 lb dumbbell in the *opposite* hand from the side you are leaning.

Stretches

Remember that in order for stretches to be safe and effective, your muscles first need to be warmed by vigorous movement. It is, therefore, best to do them after you have been training your aerobic fitness/strength/endurance.

Your ability to get into most positions for stretching specific muscles depends upon a number of factors. These include your ability to balance, limiting influences of specific health conditions, flexibility of surrounding muscles and your strength. The stretches below have been categorized as Levels 1, 2, 3, and 4, but that does not always mean that they require greater flexibility in the specific muscle in question. It may be that they require more balance or greater flexibility in surrounding muscles. You may find that for you personally, some of the Levels 3 and 4 are easier than Levels 1 or 2. The most important thing is that you find stretch positions that suit you. You need to be able to relax into the positions without straining.

Hold all stretches for a minimum of ten seconds to maintain your range of movement. If you want to increase your flexibility, then you need to relax into them for a minimum of 20–30 seconds, preferably longer. Always move into and come out of stretches slowly. Stretching should never be painful. Only take your muscles to a point where you can feel them stretching. Inhale before each stretch and exhale as you ease into it. Once in the stretch, return to regular easy breathing.

CALF (GASTROCNEMIUS)
Muscles stretched: Calves (gastrocnemius and soleus).
Where to feel the stretch: In the calf of your back leg.

Level 1
Starting position: Stand upright facing a wall, at a distance from it that just allows you to place your palms flat against it when stretching your arms out in front of you. Stand with your feet hip-distance apart and facing forwards.

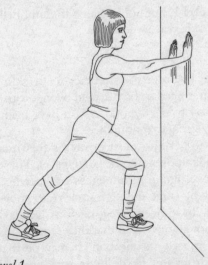

Calf Stretch Level 1

Stretching position: Lean into the wall. Take one leg as far back behind you as you can, while still keeping the foot flat on the floor. Allow the knee of your supporting leg to bend as you do so. Repeat with the other leg.

Essential technique:

- Both feet should be facing forwards; do not allow the back foot to turn outwards
- Keep your abdominals pulled in; do not allow your abdomen to drop forwards or your bottom to stick out behind you.

Level 2

The same as Level 1, but facing a chair and holding onto the seat of it so that you can go further into the stretch.

NB: To ensure that the chair is not going to slide away from you, causing you to fall, place it against a wall.

Level 3

Starting position: Stand upright with both feet on one step of a staircase. Hold onto the banister for support with the hand

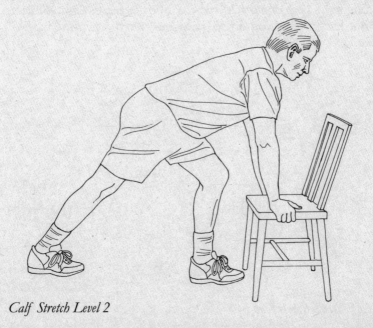

Calf Stretch Level 2

nearest to it, (or standing on a low platform, holding onto a wall for support).

Stretching position: Place the ball of your right foot on the edge of the step and then, bending the knee of the left leg, allow the heel of the right foot to drop down below the level of the step. Repeat on the other leg.

Essential technique:

- Both feet should be facing forwards
- Keep your weight over your front leg
- Keep your abdominals pulled in; do not allow your abdomen to drop forwards or your bottom to stick out behind you.

Level 4

Starting position: Get on your hands and knees on a mat, with your knees under your hips, and your hands under your shoulders. Tuck your toes under so that the pads of your toes are in contact with the floor. Pull in your abdominals firmly, then partially straighten your legs, lifting your bottom up towards the ceiling.

Stretching position: Fully straighten your right leg, pressing your right heel down towards the floor. Keep a slight bend in your left knee as you do so. Feel the stretch down the back of

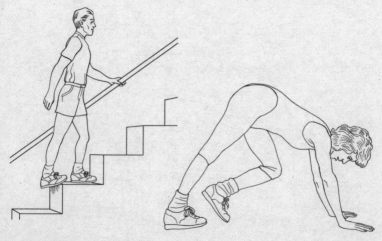

Calf Stretch Levels 3 and 4

your right calf. Hold, and then release by allowing your right heel to rise up off the floor and your right knee to bend slightly. Repeat on the other side by fully straightening your left leg, pressing your left heel down towards the floor, while your right knee remains slightly bent. Hold, and then bend both knees before returning to the starting position.

Essential technique:

- Do not lock out your elbows
- Relax the crown of your head towards the floor, and look at your feet, as you perform the stretches
- Keep your abdominals pulled in firmly throughout.

FRONT OF THIGH (QUADRICEPS)

Level 1
Starting position: Lie on your right side on a mat with a pillow, or your right arm, supporting your head. Flex at the knees and hips.
Stretching position: Using your left hand, loop a scarf around your left ankle and then use it to draw your left heel towards your left buttock. Slowly straighten your left hip until you feel a gentle stretch in the front of your left thigh. Repeat on the other side, stretching your right thigh.
Essential technique:

- Keep the shin of the leg you are stretching behind the thigh; do not pull your lower leg out sideways twisting your knee
- Keep your abdominals pulled in; do not arch your back.

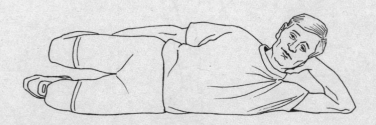

Quadriceps Stretch Level 1

Level 2
The same as Level 1, but without the use of the scarf (directly hold onto your ankle) and try to be less flexed at the hips.

Level 3
Starting position: Stand facing a wall. Place your left hand on the wall for support. Lift out of your hips by lengthening your spine. Lift your right knee up so that you can grab hold of your ankle with your right hand.
Stretching position: Keeping hold of your ankle, slowly lower your left thigh until you feel a stretch in the front of it. Repeat on the other side, stretching your right thigh.

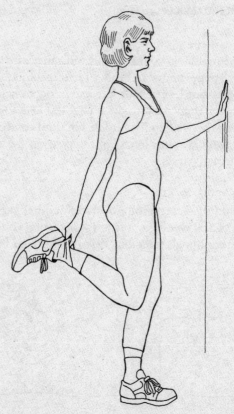

Quadriceps Stretch Level 3

Essential technique:

- Keep your abdominals pulled in; do not allow your back to arch or your bottom to stick out behind you
- Keep the shin of the leg you are stretching behind the thigh; do not pull the lower leg out sideways, twisting the knee
- Lift up out of the supporting hip; do not sink down into it
- Keep the knee of the supporting leg very slightly flexed; do not lock it out.

Level 4

Starting position: Lie face down on a mat with your forehead resting on the back of your right hand. Bend your left knee up towards your bottom and grab hold of the ankle with your left hand.

Stretching position: Holding your left ankle, slowly push your left hip down into the mat. Repeat on the other side, stretching the front of your right thigh.

Essential technique:

- Keep the shin of the leg you are stretching behind the thigh; do not pull the lower leg out sideways, twisting the knee.

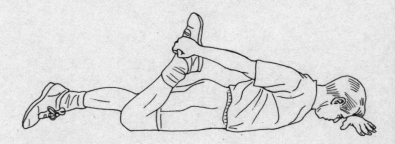

Quadriceps Stretch Level 4

BACK OF THIGH (HAMSTRINGS)

Level 1

Starting position: Place a chair with its back against a wall to ensure it will not slide away behind you. Sit upright on it, towards the edge, making sure that it is the appropriate height to put your knees at a right angle. Place your feet flat on the floor and hip-distance apart.

Stretching position: Slide one foot out in front of you along the floor until the leg is straight at the knee, but not locked. Place your hands on the tops of your thighs for support. Incline slightly forwards from the hips while simultaneously tilting your pelvis so that your abdomen tilts downwards and your tailbone lifts up behind you. Once you can feel the stretch in the back of your thigh on the leg that is straight, there is no need to incline any further forward. Simply hold the stretch, then swap the positions of the legs and stretch out your other leg.

Essential technique:

- The effectiveness of this stretch depends upon the tilting of the pelvis. Done correctly, the degree that you need to flex forward from the hips is only slight

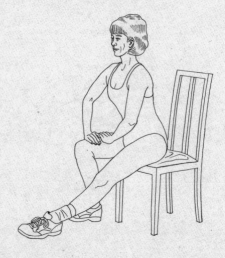

Hamstring Stretch Level 1

- Keep your back long. If you sit collapsed down into your spine, you will not be able to achieve the correct tilting of the pelvis
- As you incline forwards, use your hands on your thighs to provide some support
- Look straight ahead as you perform the stretch.

Level 2

Starting position: Place a low chair or stool against a wall. Position yourself with the wall on your right, and the stool just in front of you. Hold onto the wall for support with your right hand. Bend your left knee and place your right foot on the stool. Place your left hand on the top of your left thigh.

Stretching position: Straighten your right leg, sticking your bottom out behind you until you feel a stretch down the back of your right thigh. If you are unable to straighten your leg then the stool is too high for your current level of flexibility. Hold, then place your right foot back on the floor and change sides to stretch your left leg.

Essential technique:

- Ensure that the knee of your supporting leg remains in alignment with your ankle; do not let it roll inwards

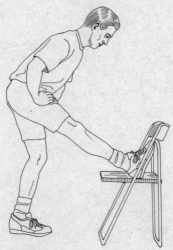

Hamstring Stretch Level 2

- Do not press down with your hands on the thigh or knee of the straight leg
- The effectiveness of this stretch depends upon the tilting of the pelvis (sticking your bottom out). Done correctly, the degree that you need to lean forward from the hips is only slight.

Level 3 Lying supine

Starting position: Lie on your back on a mat with your knees bent up and your feet flat on the floor. Place your feet hip-distance apart. Draw your right knee in towards your chest, holding onto the back of the thigh with both hands.

Stretching position: Slowly begin to straighten your right leg by taking your right foot towards the ceiling. You are unlikely to get your leg fully straight, so just straighten it as far as you need to in order to feel a stretch down the back of the thigh. Hold, and then slowly lower the leg back down to the starting position. Repeat with the left leg.

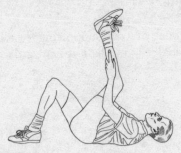

Hamstring Stretch Level 3

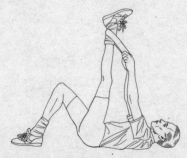

Hamstring Stretch Level 3 Alternative

Essential technique:

- If you are straining to hold your thigh, causing your shoulders to lift off the floor and your head to drop back, use a scarf to wrap around your thigh and hold it with that instead
- At no time should your buttocks lose contact with the floor
- Ensure the leg that you are not stretching remains bent up at the knee with the foot flat on the floor.

Level 4

Starting position: Sit upright on the floor with one leg straight out in front of you and the other slightly to the side with the knee bent. The knee and toes of your straight leg should be facing the ceiling. Place your hands on the thigh of your straight leg.

NB: If you cannot sit on the floor in this way, then this position is too advanced for you.

Stretching position: Lift up out of your hips, lengthen your spine, and lift your chest up and forward. Slowly lean forward over your straight leg, sticking your bottom out behind you as you do so, until you feel a stretch down the back of the thigh.

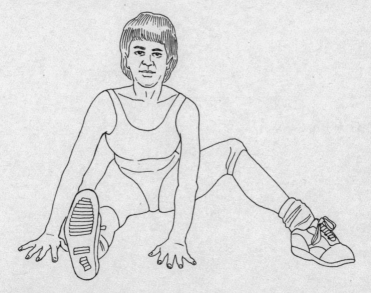

Hamstring Stretch Level 4

NB: If you are so flexible that you are coming a long way forward before you feel the stretch, then place your hands on the floor either side of your straight leg to support yourself. Hold, and then swap leg positions and stretch the other one.

Essential technique:

- Look straight ahead, not down, throughout the exercise
- Keep your shoulders back and down. *Do not round your shoulders or upper back*
- Do not attempt to reach down your leg with your hands.

FRONT OF HIP (HIP FLEXORS)

Level 1

Starting position: Sit with your left buttock on the right-side edge of a chair, with your left foot flat on the floor and your knee at a right angle. Grasp the left side of the chair seat with your left hand to support yourself, and place your right hand on your left thigh. Allow your right knee to hang down towards the floor so that your right thigh is vertical.

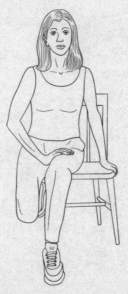

Hip Flexor Stretch Level 1

Stretching position: Slide your right foot back along the floor behind you until you feel a stretch in the front of your right hip. Hold, and then return to the starting position before sitting on the other side of the chair and stretching out your left hip.

Essential technique:

• Keep your abdominals pulled in throughout
• Maintain an upright sitting posture; do not leaning forward.

Level 2

Starting position: Standing upright, place your feet hip-distance apart and facing forwards. If necessary, hold onto the back of a chair for support. Take a large step back behind you with your right leg, placing the ball of the foot on the floor. Place both your hands on your left thigh for support. Bend both knees, keeping your weight evenly distributed over both feet.

Stretching position: Tilt your pelvis by pushing your pubic bone forwards and tucking your tailbone underneath you as far as you can. Feel the stretch in the front of the right hip. (If you have difficulty feeling the stretch, you may need to take your

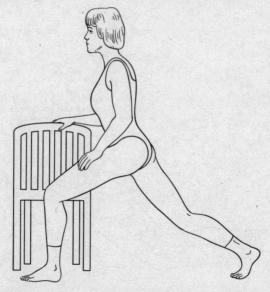

Hip Flexor Stretch Level 2

right leg further back and/or achieve a greater pelvic tilt.) Hold, and then return to the starting position before turning to face the other way and repeating the stretch on the other side.

Essential technique:

- Maintain an upright posture with your upper body throughout the exercise. Do not lean forwards or backwards
- Ensure your front knee is over your ankle and not in front of it or rolling inwards
- Keep your abdominals pulled in to support your spine.

Level 3

Starting position: Go into a Level 2 front lunge as described on page 147. This time allow your back knee to go all the way to the floor. Place your hands on the floor either side of your front leg.

Stretching position: Keeping your front knee over the ankle, slide your back knee along the floor away behind you until you feel a stretch in the front of the hip.

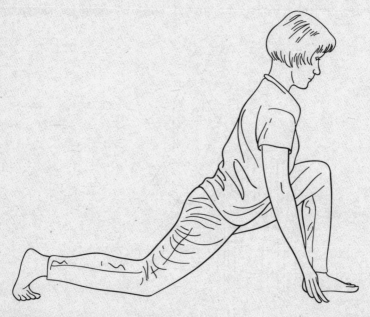

Hip Flexor Stretch Level 3

Essential technique:

- Do not let your front knee extend further forwards than the ankle
- Keep your legs hip-distance apart
- Keep your abdominals pulled in throughout the exercise to support your spine.

Level 4
The same as Level 3, but with your hands resting on your front thigh, your back upright, and looking straight ahead.

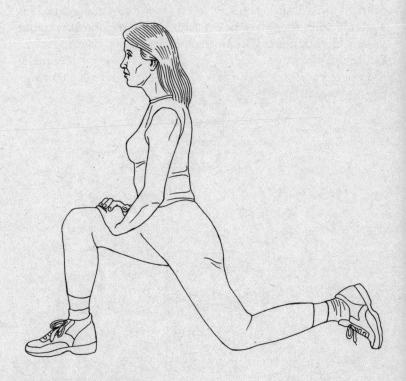

Hip Flexor Stretch Level 4

INNER THIGH (ADDUCTORS)

Level 1

Starting position: Place the back of a chair against a wall. Sit upright towards the edge of the chair with your feet flat on the floor and slightly turned out. Take your thighs as wide apart as you can while keeping your knees above your ankles. Do *not* let your knees roll inwards.

Stretching position: Hold onto the insides of your thighs, gently easing them a little further apart, until you feel a stretch on the insides of your thighs.

Essential technique:

* Keep your shoulders down and back. Do not allow your shoulders or upper back to round.

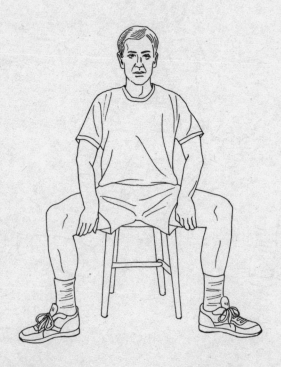

Inner Thigh Stretch Level 1

Level 2

Starting position: Stand upright. Place your feet twice as wide apart as your hips. Turn your right foot so that it is slightly, and comfortably, turned out. Turn your left foot to face directly forwards.

Stretching position: Keeping your left knee straight, and both hips facing forwards, bend your right knee towards the toes of your right foot until you feel a stretch on the inside of your left thigh. Hold, and then return to the starting position. Repeat the stretch on the other leg.

NB: If you cannot feel the stretch, then take your legs wider apart. If you need to, hold onto the back of a chair or use a wall for support.

Essential technique:

- Maintain an upright posture throughout the stretch. Do not lean forwards
- Keep your weight evenly distributed over both hips. Do not allow one hip to swing out to the side
- Ensure both hips face forwards towards the chair throughout.

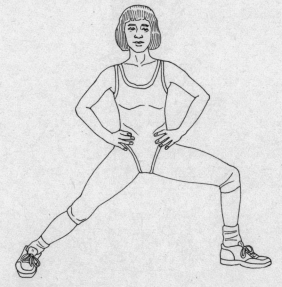

Inner Thigh Stretch Level 2

Level 3

Starting position: Sit upright on a mat with your knees bent, soles of your feet together, and knees relaxed outwards. Grasp hold of your feet or ankles and place your elbows on the insides of your knees.

Stretching position: Gently ease your knees lower to the floor by applying gentle downward pressure with your elbows.

Essential technique:

• Keep your shoulders back and down. Do not allow your shoulders or upper back to round
• Maintain a straight back, even when leaning forwards
• Keep your chest lifted and avoid looking down.

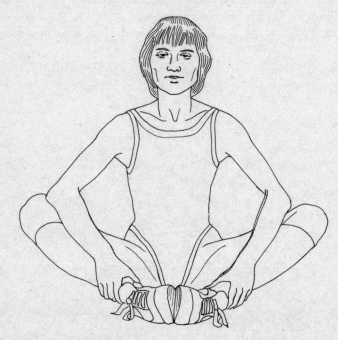

Inner Thigh Stretch Level 3

Level 4

Starting position: Sit upright on the floor with your legs in a straddled position. Your knees and toes should be facing the ceiling. Place your hands on the floor in front of you. Lengthen your neck and look forwards keeping your back straight.

Stretching position: Incline forwards slightly from the hips until you feel a stretch on the insides of your thighs. If you find yourself coming a long way forwards before you feel the stretch, then you need to take your legs further apart.

Essential technique:

- Keep your hands behind you, or resting on the floor just in front of you
- Do not attempt to reach down your legs, or touch your toes, with your hands
- Ensure that your knees and toes face the ceiling throughout the stretch.

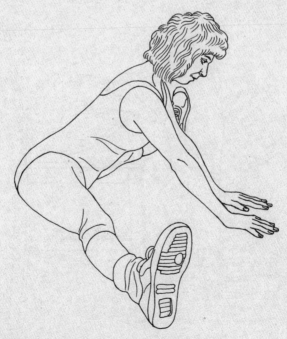

Inner Thigh Stretch Level 4

BACK (ERECTOR SPINAE)

Level 1

Starting position: Sit in a chair that places your knees at a right angle when your feet are on the floor. If the chair is too high for you to do this, place a cushion under your feet. Place your hands on your thighs.

Stretching position: Slowly lower your chin to your chest and then roll down, one vertebrae at a time, until you have brought your forehead as close as you can towards your knees without straining. Hold, and then slowly curl back up, bringing your chin up last.

Essential technique:

- Support yourself with your hands on your thighs throughout the movement
- Inhale before you begin and exhale as you roll down.

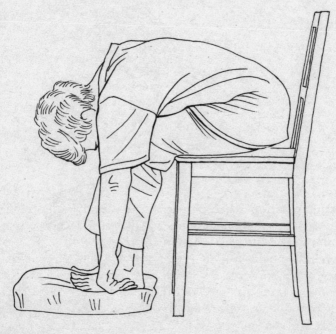

Back Stretch Level 1

Level 2

Starting position: On your hands and knees on a mat. Place your knees under your hips and your hands under your shoulders. Your fingers should be facing forwards.

Stretching position: Pulling in your abdominals, arch your back up as if you were a cat stretching, letting the crown of your head drop down towards the floor as you do so. Hold, and then relax back to the starting position.

Essential technique:

- Inhale before you go into the stretch and exhale as you arch your back. Once in position, breathe naturally
- Be sure to let the crown of your head drop towards the floor, otherwise you may experience discomfort in your neck.

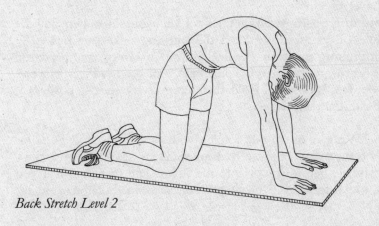

Back Stretch Level 2

Level 3

Starting position: Kneel on a mat, with your bottom resting on your heels. You may prefer to place a small cushion between your bottom and heels for extra comfort.

Stretching position: Using your arms to support yourself as you go, flex forwards from the hips, bringing your forehead down until it touches the floor in front of you. (If you cannot bring your forehead all the way to the ground, then place a pillow in front of you and rest your head on that.) Extend your arms along the floor in front of you.

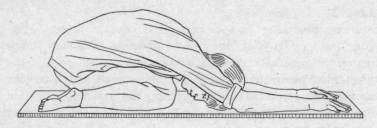

Back Stretch Level 3

Essential technique:

- Inhale before you go into the stretch and then exhale as you round forwards. Once in position, relax and breathe naturally.

Level 4
Starting position: Sit on the floor with your knees bent and the soles of your feet together. Hold onto your ankles, or toes.
Stretching position: Leading with the crown of your head, roll forwards, rounding your spine until your forehead is as close to your feet as possible. Hold, then return to the starting position.
Essential technique:

- Do not strain, or pull forcibly with your hands; only go as far as the muscles in your back are willing to stretch
- Inhale before you go into the stretch and then exhale as you round forwards. Once in position, relax and breathe naturally.

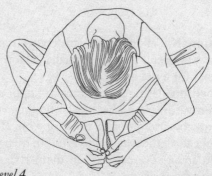

Back Stretch Level 4

FRONT OF CHEST (PECTORALS)

Level 1
Starting position: Stand upright with your weight evenly distributed over both feet. Place your hands on your bottom.
Stretching position: Maintaining an upright posture, press your elbows back behind you until you feel a stretch across the front of your chest.
Essential technique:

- Pull in your abdominals before you go into the stretch
- Avoid tipping forwards from the hips
- Do not arch your back.

Level 2
Starting position: Sit upright towards the edge of a chair. Reach behind you and grasp the chair back at about waist height.
Stretching position: Lift your chest up and forwards until you feel a stretch across the front of your chest. You might need to

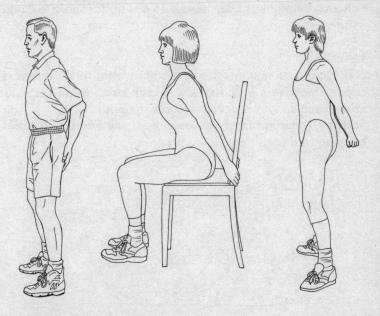

Chest Stretch Levels 1, 2 and 3

tip forwards slightly from the hips in order to achieve this. If it helps, think of yourself as a figurehead on the bow of a ship!
Essential technique:

- Pull in your abdominals before you go into the stretch
- Avoid arching your back
- Do not lock out your elbows
- Keep your shoulders down and relaxed.

Level 3
Starting position: Stand upright with your feet hip-distance apart and your abdominal muscles pulled in. Clasp your hands together behind you, or hold the opposite wrist.
Stretching position: Slowly lift your arms up behind you until you feel a stretch across the front of your chest.
Essential technique:

- Avoid arching your back
- Do not lock out your elbows
- Remain upright as you stretch; do not tip forwards from the hips.

Level 4
NB: Do not attempt this stretch if you have any of the following conditions: severe kyphosis, lower back pain, arthritis in your knees, neck, or lower back, or severe osteoporosis.
Starting position: Lie face down on a mat. Bend both knees, bringing your heels towards your bottom.

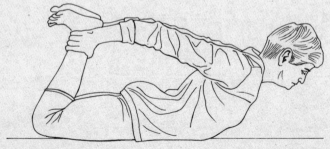

Chest Stretch Level 4

Stretching position: Reach round behind you and grasp hold of your ankles. Lift your chest up and forwards, keeping your thighs and knees on the floor. If you do not feel a stretch across the front of your chest, then push your feet away from you to increase the stretch.

Essential technique:

- Do not allow your knees or thighs to lift off the floor
- Keep your shins in alignment with your thighs
- Do not strain.

BACK OF UPPER ARM (TRICEPS)

Level 1

Starting position: Sit upright in a chair, with your feet flat on the floor. Place your right arm, with it held straight, across in front of your upper chest. Place your left hand on the back of your upper right arm.

Stretching position: Apply gentle pressure with your left hand until you feel a slight stretch down the back of your right upper arm and shoulder. Hold and then release, before repeating on the other side.

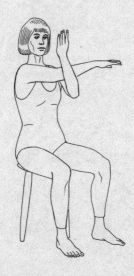

Triceps Stretch Level 1

Essential technique:

- Keep your shoulders down and back; do not hunch them
- Keep your neck long.

Level 2

Starting position: Sit upright in a chair with your feet flat on the floor. Place your right hand on the back of your neck. Place your left hand on the underside of your upper right arm.

Stretching position: Maintaining an upright posture, apply gentle pressure with your left hand to assist your right hand in reaching as far down between your shoulder blades as possible. Hold, and then release before repeating on the other side.

Essential technique:

- Avoid hunching your shoulders
- Keep your neck long
- Maintain an upright posture throughout the exercise; do not tip forwards.

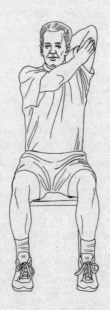

Triceps Stretch Level 2

Level 3

The same as Level 2, but this time taking your left arm overhead and placing the left hand on the right *elbow*.

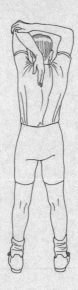

Triceps Stretch Level 3

Level 4

Starting position: Stand upright with your feet hip-distance apart. Holding a scarf in your right hand, place your right hand on the back of your neck. Reach behind you with your left hand and grab hold of the other end of the scarf.

Stretching position: Gradually start to walk the fingers of your right hand along the scarf towards your left hand, until you feel a stretch down the back of your right upper arm. The goal is to eventually be able to join hands.

Essential technique:

- Keep your abdominals pulled in throughout the exercise
- Prevent your back arching and your bottom from sticking out behind you by lifting your pubic bone up towards your belly button
- Do not strain

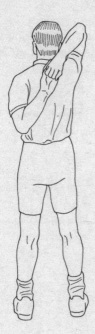

Triceps Stretch Level 4

- Keep your neck long and your shoulders down and back
- Maintain an upright stance; do not lean backwards.

SIDE OF TORSO (INTERNAL OBLIQUES)

Level 1
Starting position: Sit upright in a chair, with your feet flat on the floor. Place your right hand on the seat of the chair.
Stretching position: With your left arm, reach straight up above your head towards the ceiling, keeping both buttocks in contact with the chair, until you feel a gentle stretch down the left-hand side of your torso. Hold, and then return to the starting position. Repeat on the other side.
Essential technique:

- Maintain an upright posture throughout; do not lean forwards or backwards.

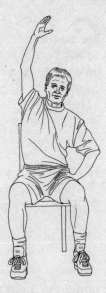

Side Stretch Level 1

Level 2

Starting position: Sit upright in a chair with your feet slightly wider apart than the chair legs. Place your right hand on the right side of the chair seat. Pull your abdominals in firmly.

Stretching position: Keeping both buttocks in contact with the chair, lift up out of your hips and lengthen your spine before leaning directly over to the right. Use your right arm to support yourself, allowing it to bend at the elbow as you lean towards it. Only go as far as you need to feel a gentle stretch down the left-hand side of your torso. Hold, and then return to the starting position. Repeat on the other side.

Essential technique:

- Do not lean forwards or backwards
- Keep both buttocks in contact with the chair throughout the exercise
- Keep your knees above your ankles; do not let them roll inwards
- Ensure that you lift your torso upwards before you attempt to lean over to the side.

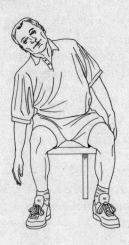

Side Stretch Level 2

Level 3

Starting position: Sit upright in a chair with your feet slightly wider apart than the chair legs. Place your right hand on your right knee.

Stretching position: With your left arm, reach straight up above your head towards the ceiling, keeping both buttocks in contact with the chair as you do so. Pull in your abdominals and then slowly lean over sideways to the left, taking your left arm with

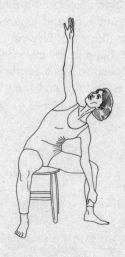

Side Stretch Level 3

you. Allow your right hand to slide down your shin as you lean into the stretch. Lean as far as you need to, supporting yourself with your right arm, until you feel a stretch down the left side of your torso. Hold, and then return to the starting position. Repeat on the other side.

Essential technique:

• Keep your knees above your ankles; do not let them roll inwards
• Do not lean forwards or backwards
• Ensure that you lift your torso upwards, by reaching towards the ceiling with your arm, before you attempt to lean over to the side.

Level 4

Starting position: Stand upright with your feet twice as wide apart as your hips. Bend slightly at the knees. Place your right hand on your right hip for support. Lengthen your spine and then reach straight up towards the ceiling with your left hand.

Stretching position: When you can reach no higher, slowly lean over the right side bringing your left arm with you. Use your right arm to support you. Lean over as far as you need to feel a stretch down the left side of your torso. Hold, and then return to the starting position before repeating on the other side.

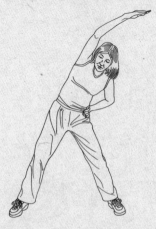

Side Stretch Level 4

Essential technique:

- Make sure your knees are over your ankles and not rolling inwards
- Keep both knees equally bent throughout
- Ensure that your bottom is not stuck out behind you
- *Do not allow your hips to swing out to one side; keep your weight central*
- Keep your abdominals very firmly pulled in throughout.

ACROSS TORSO (EXTERNAL OBLIQUES)

Level 1
Starting position: Sit upright towards the edge of a chair. Place your knees and feet together. Place your hands on the outside of your right thigh.
Stretching position: Lifting up and out of your pelvis and lengthening your spine, rotate from your waist so that your chest turns to the right. Use your hands to apply gentle pressure against the outside of your thigh, helping you to make the fullest rotation that you can comfortably achieve. Hold, and then return to the starting position before repeating on your left side.

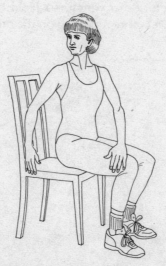

Oblique Stretch Level 1

Essential technique:

- Keep both buttocks firmly in contact with the chair throughout the exercise
- Keep your shoulders relaxed and down
- By keeping your chin above the centre of your chest, ensure that the rotation is coming from your waist and not just your neck

Level 2

Starting position: Lie on your back on a mat, with your knees bent up and your feet flat on the floor. Keep your knees and ankles together. Place a plump pillow or cushion on the floor to your right, level with your thighs. Relax your arms out along the floor at shoulder height.

Stretching position: Pull in your abdominals firmly and then, keeping your toes in contact with the floor, slowly lower both knees down onto the pillow. Once your knees are in contact with the pillow, relax all your muscles and feel the stretch diagonally across the left side of your torso. Hold, and then pull in your abdominals again before returning to the starting position. Move the pillow to your left and then repeat the stretch on the other side.

Essential technique:

- Whenever your legs are moving, your abdominals need to be pulled in firmly.

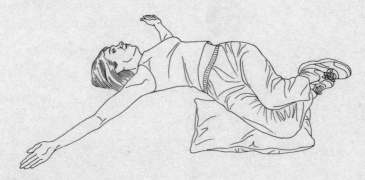

Oblique Stretch Level 2

Level 3
The same as Level 2, but without the pillow.

Level 4
Starting position: Sit upright on the floor with both legs straight out in front of you, with your knees and toes uppermost. Place your right foot on the floor to the outside of your left knee, keeping it snugly close to the knee. Place your right hand directly behind you on the floor close to your tailbone, with your fingers pointing away from you. Place your left hand on the outside of your right knee.

Stretching position: Lifting up and out of your pelvis and lengthening your spine, rotate from your waist so that your chest turns to the right. Use your left hand to apply gentle pressure against the outside of your knee, helping you to make the fullest rotation that you can comfortably achieve. Hold, and then return to the starting position before repeating on your left side.

Essential technique:

- Maintain an upright posture, do not lean back from the hips
- Keep both buttocks firmly in contact with the chair throughout the exercise
- Keep your shoulders relaxed and down
- Ensure that the rotation is coming from your waist and not just your neck, by keeping your chin above the centre of your chest.

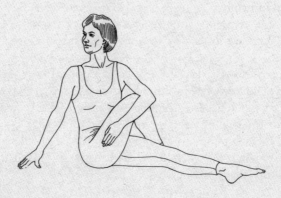

Oblique Stretch Level 4

Chapter 6
Helping Your Body Heal with Exercise

The full healing powers of the human body are beyond the understanding of medical science. Although a bone, when broken, can be immobilized or realigned by intervention, only your body can perform the necessary processes for that bone to mend. No type of exercise can actually perform any healing for you, but it can provide your body with the opportunity it needs to heal itself and enhance its efforts to do so.

For example, it is dynamic movement of your body that enables lymphatic fluids to circulate and fulfil their roles in healing on many levels. Movement of your joints enables synovial fluid to be produced within them, making it possible for brittle and dehydrated articular cartilage to regain its sponginess. Muscle mass dictates your metabolic rate, governing the speed at which all anabolic (building up) and catabolic (breaking down) processes occur. In the absence of cardio-respiratory fitness, insufficient quantities of blood and oxygen reach your cells, severely impeding all your body's attempts to heal and repair its damaged tissues. Without movement, your bone-building cells fail to be stimulated into action, crippling your body's attempts to replace lost bone mass. These are just a few examples of how exercise is vital to healing.

In many cases, a lack of exercise is one of the causes of a specific condition of ill health. In some cases it is even the primary cause and, in a few cases, the sole cause. Here we are going to take a look at the role of exercise in helping your body to heal from four of the most common conditions amongst people who are in the second half of their lives: arthritis, cardiovascular disease, obesity and osteoporosis.

Arthritis

The word arthritis comes from the Greek words *aurton* (joint) and *itis* (inflammation). There many different types of arthritis, but the most common are rheumatoid (RA) and osteo (OA). The causes, physical progressions and implications for RA and OA are considerably different from each other.

Osteoarthritis (OA)

This is the most common form of arthritis, affecting approximately 80 per cent of people over the age of 65. It is twice as common amongst women as men. Osteoarthritis is confined to the joints and the soft tissues immediately surrounding them. For a better understanding of this condition, let's take a moment for a spot of revision.

The junctions where two or more of your bones meet are known as joints. Not all the joints in your body move. The many different bones that make up your skull, for example, complete their formation during infancy and then remain relatively immobile. All freely movable joints such as elbows, knees and hips, are encased within a special capsule (synovial capsule). The purpose of this capsule is to provide the joint with lubrication and protection. In order to prevent bones from grinding directly against each other, the ends are covered with cartilage, a soft durable tissue that helps bone surfaces to glide smoothly on contact with each other. This cartilage also acts as a cushion to absorb shock. It is through the synovial capsule and cartilage pads working together that joints are kept healthy and functional. Each time joints are moved, the lining of the synovial capsule becomes stimulated to produce a lubricant (synovial fluid), which is then soaked up by the cartilage pads. Only when engorged with fluid can the pads fulfil their role as shock absorbers and properly cushion the bone ends.

A sedentary lifestyle leads to inadequate stimulation of the synovial capsule and a consequent lack of synovial fluid production. The consequence is that the articular cartilage quickly becomes dehydrated and eventually begins to disintegrate. It is then no longer able to function as a protective cushion for the bone ends and so they become damaged.

Healthy cartilage does not contain nerve fibres. In order to restore damaged cartilage, however, the body must grow nerves that will extend into it. This results in painful joints and a tendency for a person to become even more sedentary. The result is a downward spiral of further dehydration, disintegration and damage. Once the protective cartilage has been lost to a significant degree, the body takes additional action to protect the bone ends by forming bony spurs (osteophytes) on the articulating surfaces. The result is a considerable increase in pain and loss of movement range.

In addition, a very high percentage of joint stiffness results from changes within the soft tissues of the synovial capsule. It is for this reason that appropriate exercise is vital in the management of this condition.

Excess Strain on Joints

Although leading a sedentary lifestyle is a primary cause of osteoarthritis, the excessive overuse of joints, especially if this involves weight-bearing and/or direct trauma, can also result in degeneration of cartilage and damaged painful joints. For example, years of regularly running long distances on hard roads while overfat will be paid for in joint health. For people of a healthy body weight, running and jogging are excellent and natural ways to exercise. The surfaces most people run on, however, are not natural. Roads lack shock-absorbing qualities and usually have a camber that consistently and repeatedly throws the hips out of alignment at one specific angle. Ideally, running should be done on soft ground that reduces the impact on the joints and naturally undulates in a variety of ways to avoid repetitive stress injuries. If you run or jog regularly, you must invest in a good pair of shoes designed specifically for the job. Running with the correct technique involves the heel striking the ground first and taking most of the impact. Good shoes should therefore have plenty of protection at the heel, as well as feel comfortable and have a flexible sole.

If your preferred form of exercise is attending exercise-to-music classes, avoid lengthy bouts of high impact work, especially if you are overfat or do not have suitable shoes for the floor surface. A good teacher will offer low impact alternatives. Remember – when jogging or springing on the spot, it is mechanically impossible to land heels first! Impact must be taken through the ball of the foot and then transmitted to the heel. Although the body is designed to cope with this mode of landing, it is unnatural to perform such a movement for the extended number of repetitions typical in many exercise-to-music classes.

When OA is caused by previous injuries (such as joint fractures), excessive force or overuse from sports or occupational hazards, it is classified as secondary OA. Osteoarthritis that exists without a clinically recognized cause is referred to as primary. Both types of OA can affect any joint, but the hip, knee and finger joints are the most common sites. When the weight-bearing joints (hips and knees) are affected, the result is inevitably reduced mobility, which in turn exacerbates the condition. In addition, in an attempt to avoid pain and compensate for reduced range of movement, the afflicted person will tend habitually to adopt a compromised posture and way of moving. This causes mild to severe biomechanical misalignment of the joints, damaging them further.

Symptoms and signs of OA include swelling, creaking and inflammation of the joints as well as reduced ranges of movement and, eventually, joint deformities. Early morning stiffness is typical with OA – it tends to wear off later in the day. Joint stiffness can be made worse by long periods of sitting.

Rheumatoid Arthritis (RA)

This condition is a chronic inflammatory disease, affecting all aspects of the synovial capsules that encase the freely movable joints. Unlike osteoarthritis, RA also affects many other aspects of the body and is notorious for demonstrating flare-up phases and periods of relief. It is classified in medical terms as an autoimmune condition. Rheumatoid arthritis is three times more common in women than in men, and typically starts between the ages of 30 and 40. In 50 per cent of cases, the hips are affected.

Symptoms of RA include joint pain at night and first thing in the morning – sometimes lasting for several hours. Fatigue and a general malaise typically accompany these symptoms. Signs include swelling of the soft tissues, tenderness of the joints on pressure or movement, reduced ranges of movement and eventual deformity of the joints. Manifestations of the condition not affecting the joints include carpal tunnel syndrome, sensory loss, muscular weakness, anaemia, and lung and spleen problems.

Approaches taken in an attempt to treat arthritis include physiotherapy, occupational therapy, orthotics (aids and appliances), surgery (including joint replacements) and drugs. Drugs commonly used are salicylates, nonsteroidal anti-inflammatory drugs and intra-articular steroids. In Appendix 1 you will find information regarding the implications of taking these drugs. If you suffer from RA or OA, one of the most important things you can do for your joints is to shed excess body weight. The reduced movement common to arthritis typically leads to weight gain, which only compounds the problem. The impact of each step you take while walking can be several times your body weight, hence this can be reduced by nine to 15 lbs (4 to 6.5 kg) for every three lbs (1.25 kg) of body weight you lose. If you suffer from RA, never exercise joints that are experiencing a flare up of pain, redness and warmth. Likewise, rest rather than exercise if you have a fever or an infection of any description.

How Exercise Helps Arthritis
Overall, the golden rule is that the less you use your joints, the weaker and stiffer they become. General movement of arthritic joints has been shown to reduce congestive swelling and therefore allow a greater range of movement. Simply keeping mobile and avoiding extensive periods of time spent sitting is greatly helpful. There are, however, specific things you can do to reduce pain and the likelihood of further deterioration.

Posture
If you suffer from either OA or RA, it is probable that your posture will become more flexed the greater your discomfort. Unfortunately any compromise in your posture will further damage your joints. Refer back to Chapter Three to revise what constitutes good posture when sitting, standing, and walking. Then make a point of observing your posture whenever you get the chance – in full-length mirrors, your reflection in shop windows and in photographs. Much of your postural alignment will be dictated by your psychological viewpoint. Developing a

sense of renewed pride in your appearance, and a heightened pursuit of grace, can result in you looking ten years younger and can pave the way for rejuvenation of your joints.

Mobilizing

Mobilization exercises, as described with reference to warm ups in Chapter Four, are a vital form of movement for arthritic joints. By regularly taking the joints through the limits of their pain-free range, mobility can be preserved and even developed over time.

When mobilizing your joints, always begin with small ranges of movement and then gradually increase them until you are moving just within the limits of your pain-free range. Remember to mobilize all your little joints too, such as the joints of your fingers. It is recommended that you take time to thoroughly mobilize your joints at least twice each day. Upon first awakening in the morning, and again before you retire for the night, are good options.

Aerobic Exercise

If you suffer from arthritis, developing your cardio-respiratory fitness will be extremely helpful. Aerobic exercise will increase the blood supply to your joints and improve your overall health. In addition, if you are carrying any excess weight, this type of exercise will play an important role in helping you to reduce it. The types of aerobic exercise most suitable for arthritic joints are those that involve minimal weight bearing. Swimming and cycling are both good examples. If swimming is your preferred choice, then the crawl is far preferable to the breaststroke. This is because the angle your knees – and to a lesser extent your hips – assume to perform the breaststroke can be stressful on the joints. Bouncing on a mini-trampoline can provide a great aerobic workout and strengthen muscles while minimizing trauma to your joint surfaces. If you take up this fun activity, be sure to begin gently by hardly leaving the bed of the trampoline. Do not attempt to bounce any higher until the muscles in your legs have become strong enough to keep your knees in good alignment as you land.

Strength Training

Significant muscle weakness is experienced by 80 per cent of people with arthritis. This is caused by the overall reduction in movement as a result of pain. The consequence of such immobility can be a 45–75 per cent loss of strength.

Strength training is vital to maintain functional ability, to provide superior support for the joints, and to increase the density of the bones. Muscles can be strengthened by either isotonic or isometric exercises. When muscles contract and bring about movement of the bones (such as when you lift your arm in the air), this is classified as isotonic exercise. When muscles contract but bring about no movement of the bones (such as when you press the palms of your hands together), it is known as isometric exercise. For joints affected by arthritis, isometric exercise can be very helpful because isometric strength is needed to hold the bones in correct alignment as you go about your day. There are, however, two primary disadvantages of this type of training.

Firstly, your functional strength will be limited to the one point, in any given range of movement, where you have practised the exercise. You will not be strong throughout the entire range of movement, but only in the one position, at the precise angle at which you train. Secondly, at the time of performing isometric work there is a considerable, although momentary, rise in your blood pressure. For this reason, if you already suffer from hypertension (high blood pressure), it is best for you not to use isometric work to increase your strength but to rely on isotonic training instead. Even if you have a moderately healthy blood pressure, it is recommended that you do not hold any isometric contractions for longer than six seconds and that you take a ten-second rest between each repetition. If you are training in sets (groups of repetitions), it is best to rest for one whole minute between each set. There is a tendency to hold your breath when doing isometric exercises, which should be avoided, as it will contribute to raising your blood pressure. Whatever approach you take to strength training, make sure that you strengthen all the major muscles groups, not just those surrounding the affected joints.

Stretching

Performing stretches at least once daily is paramount for maintaining ranges of movement. Stretching each muscle two or three times on each occasion is an excellent approach for arthritic joints. Your calves, hamstrings, lower back and the front of your shoulders are likely to be especially inflexible. Allow yourself plenty of time to get into the correct position and initiate good technique before executing each stretch. Finish off with a thorough mobilization of your joints to promote circulation and reduce stiffness.

General Advice for Arthritis Sufferers

If your joints are already to some degree arthritic, then the following guidelines will help you avoid getting worse. They can even bring about significant improvements:

- Dividing your exercise sessions up throughout the day is far preferable to intense bouts followed by hours of inactivity. Three ten-minute sessions are far more suitable for arthritis sufferers than one 30-minute session
- If your arthritis is so severe that it prevents you from walking for more than five minutes at a time, do not increase the duration of your exercise sessions more than 10 per cent per week
- Avoid all twisting or explosive movements and anything done with momentum
- Listen to your body and do not attempt to override pain
- Learn to recognize the difference between increased joint pain and muscle soreness
- Become familiar with your usual level of joint pain so that you can assess how it has changed following exercise
- If any additional soreness brought about by exercising has not disappeared two hours after you have stopped exercising, then you need to change your exercise approach
- Beware of exercising while on painkillers, as the limits of your joint's comfortable range will be masked. In this case you may end up taking your joints to extremes of movement, ones they are incapable of making without exacerbating their condition
- Find a time of day to exercise when your joints usually feel their best
- Try to walk on even ground and avoid terrain that is stony, bumpy or in any way uneven
- Wear shoes that provide significant cushioning at all times, such as trainers

- Avoid taking your joints beyond their natural ranges of flexion and extension
- Do not add force of any sort to your joints when they are in a fully flexed, or fully extended, position. For example, avoid squatting so deeply that your hips are below the height of your knees or holding a very heavy object with your knees locked out.

Being arthritic does not mean that you cannot enjoy sports and other physical activities, even though some are inappropriate as they will exacerbate your condition. In addition to swimming and cycling, table tennis, aquarobics, walking and even cross-country skiing are examples of activities in which you could safely participate. What you need to avoid is anything that throws your joints out of correct alignment (such as walking on uneven ground or skiing moguls), is explosive (such as discus, shot put or javelin) or involves a lot of lateral movements (such as squash). Pastimes that put you at risk from falling, impact or collision (such as ice-skating or football) are also unsuitable. Depending on your degree of mobility, some activities such as horse riding may require a greater range of movement than your joints can accommodate.

Two popular recreational pursuits are golf and bowls. If your knees are affected by arthritis, unless you are a truly expert player, golf is not going to be appropriate for you due to the swing involved, as it can throw your knees out of alignment. Be wary also of bowls, as the momentum transmitted to your hips and knees may be more than those joints can comfortably withstand. If tennis is your game, then get sociable and play doubles rather than singles. This way you are less likely to attempt extreme lateral movements across the court. The greatest danger in tennis for arthritic joints is the high friction that can exist between the bottoms of your feet and the court surface. This can place tremendous force laterally through your knee joints and even result in falling. Investing in a good quality pair of well-designed tennis shoes will minimize this foot-to-court friction and is a must for arthritic players.

Preventing Arthritis
Here we will explore the role of movement and the mechanical use of your body in maintaining healthy joints.

Avoid Stressing Joints

Any attempts to move joints through a range that they are not designed to make can damage the surrounding soft tissues and lead to injury. Ligaments, for example, are bands of fibrous tissue that act rather like guy ropes, securing bone to bone by attaching them where they meet. Healthy ligaments allow for a slight deviation of the joints' naturally intended ranges of movement, but they do not accommodate more profound deviations. Ligaments have minimal flexibility and a poor blood supply, which means they take a long time to heal once damaged.

Knees are notorious for being problematical. Frequently this is because the surrounding muscles have been allowed to become weak. This not only reduces the stability of these weight-bearing hinge joints, but also leaves them susceptible to misalignment, especially when bending. Whenever you bend your knees to pick something up, always be sure to keep them well turned out and moving in the direction of your toes. This is especially important if carrying a heavy weight or when landing after jumping.

Avoid activities that subject your joints to repeated stress. Aerobic 'step' exercise, for example, involves stepping repeatedly up and down from a low platform. It is a fun way to add variety to your exercise sessions and effective as an aerobic conditioner. If done to excess, however, stepping can result in repetitive stress injuries to your knees and lower back.

The best way to exercise is to take part in the widest possible range of activities. This way you will develop a broad range of fitness, while minimizing the risk of overusing any specific joint. As you get older there is a tendency for the body to slowly dehydrate, and as this happens the soft tissues surrounding your joints become more vulnerable. These tissues become far more pliable and less viscous once warmed through movement, however. Because of this it is especially important to perform a proper warm-up prior to playing sports, exercising or undertaking physically demanding tasks.

Joints are at their most vulnerable when in hyper-flexed or hyper-extended positions, especially if weight bearing at the time. This means that in order to look after your joints, care needs to be taken when performing certain activities of daily life. For example, if squatting, such as when gardening or scrubbing floors, avoid allowing your hips to drop lower than your knees. Preferably perch on a small stool or move onto your hands and knees.

Avoid Direct Injuries

An obvious aspect of preventing OA is to minimize your risk of sustaining direct injuries to your joints. Contact sports, skiing and horse riding are all examples of high-risk activities. Apart from direct acute trauma, another type of potential injury to be aware of is the accumulated effect of repetitively placing abnormal stress upon your joints. This has been shown to be a significant cause of OA. You may be surprised to learn that repetitive natural movements within the joints' intended range, such as running, do not in themselves result in damage to the joints. Due to the lateral forces and collisions involved in football, players of this game show a far greater prevalence to OA than long-distance runners. Still, it is important to run, and walk, with a heel–toe action to maximize the body's natural shock dispersal mechanisms. Seeking out natural surfaces to exercise on is also the best approach. Regular activities involving moderate impact (such as jogging and running) are, however, inappropriate if you are more than 10 per cent overfat. This is because the unnatural load on your joints can stress them to the point of damage.

Finally, whatever your age, state of health or time constraints, take time daily to put your joints gently through their naturally intended range of movement a few times. This will help to keep them lubricated, protected and healthy. Warm up properly before strenuous activities, and develop the habit of a comprehensive fitness regimen to keep the muscles around your joints strong and flexible.

Heart Disease and Hypertension

Back as recently as the late 1800s, death as a result of insufficient oxygen reaching the heart (heart attack) or the brain (stroke) was so rare that it was not mentioned in any of the medical records of that time. These days, the condition is so common that somebody dies of it every 25 seconds!

In the 1800s, people consumed only modest amounts of flesh and dairy foods as the majority of their diet was plant based. Until the invention of the combustion engine, farmers were limited in the amount of plant foods that they could physically produce in any given season. But once tractors, combine harvesters, and other machines were available, food production increased dramatically. Farmers were then able to reap such vast quantities of produce that the feeding and fattening of livestock for human consumption became a massive industry. This resulted in changing the consumption of meat and dairy products from small amounts that accompanied plant based menus into the focal point of every meal. The incidence of heart attacks and strokes has now reached epidemic proportions. Both are conditions that are almost entirely avoidable.

First, it needs to be understood that 'risk factors' and 'causes' are not the same thing. A risk factor is something that statistics have shown to be common amongst people suffering from a certain condition. A cause is a direct influence that contributes to, or is exclusively responsible for, creating the condition. Classically, age, genetics and gender are the three main factors considered to indicate a person's risk of experiencing cardiovascular disease. This can be misleading for the following reasons:

Age – atherosclerosis and arteriosclerosis are cumulative conditions and so take many years to gradually manifest. The ageing process itself does not cause cardiovascular disease.

Genetics – although it has been assumed for decades that genetics can predispose a person to cardiovascular disease, it has been demonstrated that inherited lifestyle and dietary habits are far more relevant than inherited physiological vulnerabilities.

Gender – in the past men have been statistically more at risk, but today the incidence of heart attack and stroke amongst women is almost as high as men. In fact, women are equally at risk once past menopause.

Atherosclerosis – this is the progressive build up of fatty deposits and cholesterol on the inside of the artery walls. It is caused by the consumption of saturated fats and cholesterol present in all meat, poultry, fish and dairy products. Smoking, diabetes, inactivity, stress and alcohol consumption all contribute to causing this condition.

Hypertension – this is the term used to describe an abnormally high blood pressure. This is measured as systolic pressure (pressure in the arteries during the contractile phase of each heartbeat) and diastolic pressure (pressure in the arteries when the heart muscle relaxes). Other possible causes include disorders of the kidneys or adrenal glands and coarctation of the aorta (a congenital heart defect).

Heart attack – (also known as myocardial infarction) is the sudden death of part(s) of the heart muscle. Such an event is caused by the blood supply to the heart being impeded or totally blocked. The causes of a heart attack are either the presence of atherosclerotic plaques, an embolism (blockage by something such as a segment of plaque or a clot of blood), or an aneurysm (a ruptured blood vessel).

Angina – refers to pains felt in the chest, shoulder, upper back or left arm that are evidence of the blood supply to the heart being seriously impeded.

Stroke – (also known as a cerebral infarction) describes when damage to part of the brain occurs caused by an interruption in its flow of blood or leakage of its blood supply through the walls of its blood vessels. The same dietary and lifestyle habits that cause heart attacks also cause strokes.

Ischaemic attack – describes transient moments when vision, speech, sensation or movement become impaired due to insufficient blood reaching the brain. Ischaemic attacks are a warning sign that a stroke will ensue unless action is taken to correct diet and lifestyle.

The Benefits of Regular Exercise for Cardiovascular Health

In Chapter Three, the benefits of exercises for your heart, lungs and blood vessels are described in detail. Here is a summary of the ways in which exercise is vital for keeping your heart and circulation healthy.

With regular aerobic exercise:

- The amount of blood your heart pumps out into your body each time it beats, known as your stroke volume, increases. This results in your heart not needing to beat so frequently, therefore reducing the overall workload of your heart muscle
- There is an increase in the network of the vessels that provide your heart with its own supply of blood

- The stickiness of your blood's platelets reduces, resulting in your being less likely to experience thrombosis
- Your blood pressure will gradually normalize (providing your diet is healthy)
- There is an increase in your HDL cholesterol and a reduction in your LDL count
- There is an increase in the volume of your circulating blood during each exercise session. This has a 'flushing' effect on the inside of the arteries and so helps to prevent the build up of fatty plaques
- The elasticity of your blood vessels is enhanced, making it less likely that you will suffer from an aneurysm
- You will be better able to process the physical manifestations of your psychological stress and also are more likely to be calmer
- You will be much more able to reduce excess body fat.

Notes on Posture and Stretching

Any painful experience can cause a change in posture, but this is especially true in the case of chest pain. A tendency to round the shoulders, 'cave in' in the chest and adopt a stooped posture is common. Performing the following stretches at least twice a day can be very helpful in correcting the posture and instilling a greater feeling of confidence:

- Front of chest (pectorals)
- Sides of torso (internal obliques).

(See pages 157 and 162 for the relevant exercises.)

Guidelines for Exercise if You Have High Blood Pressure

Before you do anything else, consider removing the causes of your condition. It is typically the consumption of animal flesh and dairy products that results in hypertension. By removing, or at least reducing, the inclusion of these substances in your diet you can minimize the likelihood of experiencing a heart attack or stroke in the years to come.

Guidelines for Exercise if You Are Fitted with a Pacemaker

It is likely, if you have been fitted with a pacemaker, that you have become extremely out of condition and have a very low level of fitness. The good news is that this can be reversed. With dedication and commitment, you can recondition yourself and regain your youthfulness. Progress may be slow, but remember that it is the tortoise that wins the race!

Begin with the mobility exercises described in Chapter Four, accompanied by some gentle walking of a duration and intensity that feels manageable to you. Once you can walk for 20 minutes on level ground, begin with Level 1 of the cardio-respiratory and endurance training programmes. Also introduce some gentle stretches by performing those shown for Level 1 of the flexibility-training programme.

It is very important that you do not allow yourself to become exhausted and be sure to match the time you spend exercising with an equal amount of time resting. Be patient and progress gradually.

Do not concern yourself with starting the strength-training programme until you can comfortably achieve two sets of 20 repetitions of all exercises in Level 2 of the endurance exercises.

Very importantly, if you are to experience a superior level of health it is necessary that you to take better care of your heart and blood vessels by minimising your consumption of animal fats.

Guidelines for Exercise if You Have Experienced One or More Heart Attacks in the Past

In order to avoid future vascular episodes, begin by actively removing the primary causes of heart attacks. This involves min-imizing the meat and dairy foods in your diet and avoiding all inhalation of tobacco. The fact that you have experienced one or more heart attacks in the past may or may not have significant bearing on your current fitness level. If the causes of your vascu-lar blockages have been removed and you have been investing in regular exercise, you might be fitter today than someone who has not experienced a heart attack at all.

Conversely, your heart attack may have left you untrusting and frightened of your own body, or believing that the appropriate response to such an experience is to 'take it easy' from now on.

If this is the case, then your fitness level may have deteriorated to a very low level. Provided that the causes of your heart attack have been removed and the necessary adjustments in your diet and lifestyle have been made, there is no reason why you cannot enter into the fitness programme detailed in this book, at whatever level feels comfortable for you.

Guidelines for Exercise if You Have Recently Experienced a Heart Attack

The first thing that you need to do is to prevent a future heart attack by removing the causes from your diet and lifestyle (see above). It is possible that you had a low level of fitness before your vascular episode. Even if you did not, you will have undergone substantial bed rest in the hospital. The first stage in your fitness recovery is to once again become mobile. This means performing everyday tasks such as sitting, standing, walking and stair climbing. It is also an excellent time to exercise your joints by taking them several times through their intended ranges of movement at least once a day (see Chapter Four).

During the early days of being an out-patient, continue to increase your functional capacity by taking responsibility for as many simple, non-strenuous tasks around the home and garden as you feel able. If you want to take some gentle walks outside that is excellent, but try to avoid getting cold or overheated. Performing gentle stretches will be helpful to release tension and lengthen the muscles that will have shortened during your period of bed rest.

By the time you become an intermediate out-patient, it will have been between three to eight weeks since you were discharged from hospital. Around this time, you should be ready to start going for a walk each day. Begin on level ground and gradually increase the duration of your walk before you begin to include any inclines. This is a time for rebuilding your confidence in your physical abilities and developing your body awareness. Your heart attack may have left you fearful of your own body. Providing you have gained an understanding of what caused your condition and made the appropriate changes in your diet and lifestyle, you have every reason to feel positive and in control of your health. Exercises to build up your muscular endurance can be commenced at this stage. Turn to Chapter Five and begin with Level 1 of the endurance-training programme. Listen to your body at all times and, most importantly, get plenty of rest and sleep.

When eventually you can walk for an hour and perform two sets of 20 repetitions of all the exercises in Level 1 of the endurance-training programme, you are ready to begin with Level 1 of the strength training. Before you do, ask your doctor to test your blood pressure to ensure that this type of exercise is not inappropriate for you. Remember that although the long-term effect of exercise is a reduction in blood pressure, it actually causes a rise in blood pressure at the time of performance, especially if you are training your strength. If your doctor gives you the go-ahead, then have no hesitation to begin developing this important aspect of your fitness. Simply be sure not to hold your breath as you perform the exercises.

Once your new dietary, lifestyle and exercise habits have been set in motion, the challenge is to establish them as long-term habits. All you need is education, inspiration and opportunity. The education you need is within the pages of this book. Re-reading Chapters One to Four will help you to feel confident in your choices of diet, lifestyle and exercise. Your heart attack no doubt left you inspired to do all you can to avoid such an event in the future.

Finally, if you make an authentic commitment to creating health for yourself, providence will move in and provide you with an abundance of opportunities to follow through!

Guidelines for Exercise if You Have Experienced a Stroke

The length of time that you will have been kept in hospital depends on the severity of your stroke and the portion of your brain that was affected. The diversity of the possible outcomes from strokes, and the appropriate recommendations, is far too broad to include in this book. Whatever the details of your particular case, the most important thing to do first is to remove the causes of your stroke so as not to experience another one. Admittedly, there are cases where stroke results from influences not governed by eating or lifestyle habits, such as direct traumas, surgical procedures and other rare circumstances, but these are the exceptions, not the rule.

The physiotherapists will typically continue to work with you until you are no longer showing obvious improvements. Do not assume this to be the limits of your own healing. Many people have gone on to regain significant faculties and movement abilities as a result of a dedication to continuing exercise once discharged from therapy. At the back of the book, you will find listed the contact details of organizations and support groups that will assist you in maximizing your recovery.

Angina and Ischaemic Attacks – Remember

Angina and transient ischaemic attacks are warning signs that unless you change your dietary and lifestyle habits you will go on to experience a heart attack or stroke. Although exercise is paramount in keeping your heart and blood vessels healthy, it cannot alone correct the problem, because a lack of exercise did not *cause* the problem. It is only by removing the causes and making the necessary changes in what you eat, the way you process your life experiences (stress), and, if applicable to you, your intake of tobacco smoke and alcohol, that will free you from these pains.

Obesity

There does seem to be some degree of decline in fat metabolism as people age. It is somewhat controversial whether this is caused by the ageing process itself or by the accumulation of unhealthful dietary and lifestyle practices, especially a lack of exercise. Carrying extra body fat is not healthy, as it predisposes you to:

- Cardiovascular disease
- Cancer
- Hypertension (high blood pressure)
- Diabetes (it is estimated that 80–90 per cent of type 2 diabetics are overweight)
- Stress
- Gastrointestinal disorders
- Oedema (fluid retention)
- Respiratory Ailments (including obesity hypoventilation syndrome)
- Fallen arches (flat feet)
- Osteoarthritis of the weight-bearing joints (especially the knees)

- Poor posture
- Mood swings (due to rebound hypoglycaemia)
- Low self-esteem and poor self image
- Skin burn (due to the skin rubbing together on the inner thighs and underarms).

When your body is encumbered with extra bulk, everyday movements become more challenging and fatigue is always present to some degree. The physical appearance of excess fat may be objectionable to you and when compounded by the visible processes of ageing, it can lead to reduced self-esteem. The world of slimming rides on a multi-million-pound industry of quick fixes and miracle concoctions. The typical underlying message is that for very little effort you can get massive results – provided you invest your money in THIS! The vast majority of commercial diets have an even higher price than a monetary one, because a degree of sacrificing your overall health is usually involved.

The sad truth is that most diets fail. Even those that succeed in bringing about a significant initial weight loss typically result in eventual weight gain beyond that of the original weight. One reason for this is that most people who have been 'fighting the flab' for years are acquainted with only two ways of being: they are either on a diet or eating whatever they desire as they take a break *between* diets. Few habitual dieters have ever developed an understanding, and practical familiarity, with straightforward healthy eating that will eventually take them to, and maintain, their weight-loss goals.

What people need to HEAR is the recipe for losing excess body fat. It comprises of four ingredients:

H – Healthy diet
E – Exercise
A – Addiction withdrawal
R – Release emotional dependence on food.

Healthy Diet

A healthy diet is one that:

- Provides you with the appropriate number of calories to maintain your healthy body weight

- Provides all the nutrients, in correct ratios, that your body needs
- Is minimal in health-destroying substances.

In order to identify the approximate number of calories that you need to consume in a day follow this simple calculation:

> Multiply your healthy body weight, in pounds, by 12.5.
> Add on an appropriate number of calories according to the degree that you are physically active. As a comparative guide: a one-hour walk uses about 300 calories and a one-hour run about 600. (This is only approximate, as the heavier a person's body weight the more calories they expend when exerting, but it is accurate enough for the purposes of this exercise.)
> Add this final figure onto your calculation.
> Example:
> Healthy body weight, 130 pounds $\times$ 12 = 1,625
> 1,625 + 300 (equivalent to one hour's walking) = 1,925.

Once you have ascertained the number of calories you need, the next step is to ensure that those calories are providing you with the nutrients your body needs. The greater the percentage of whole plant foods you include in your diet, the more likely this will be. Since your body needs about 10 per cent of its calories to come from fats, any food that contains more than 10 per cent of this nutrient should be eaten sparingly. (There are many books and charts available that will provide you with the fat content of various foods.) You also need only about 10 per cent of your calories to come from protein. With the exception of items such as refined sugar, oils and alcohol, most foods you eat are going to provide at least this amount. It is carbohydrate that you need the most of; about 80 per cent of your calories need to come from this nutrient.

Exercise
Without exercise, dieting alone in an attempt to lose weight can be compared to pushing a car from A to B as opposed to driving it. Aerobic exercise, muscular strength and muscular-endurance training each make an enormous contribution to any attempt to reduce body fat. If you are overfat it is especially important that

you perform a proper warm-up before exercising. There are various reasons for this, including the fact that your weight-bearing joints need special care and preparation. This means you need to thoroughly mobilize them, as described on page 88. A warm up also gives you an opportunity to pay maximal attention to your posture, which is vital if you are to perform your exercises with good technique. You need to increase the intensity of your warm up gradually, allowing your body extra time to adapt to the demands of increased activity. Keep your arms below shoulder height to begin with, so as to avoid sudden increases in your blood pressure. Once you have mobilized your joints and moved enough to feel warmer, it is a good idea to include a few very gentle stretches. The two stretches below are especially recommended, as they will enhance the posture of your upper body and your ability to breathe deeply.

- Lateral Side Stretch
- Pectoral Stretch.

See pages 162–6 and 157–9 for the relevant exercises.

Cardio-Respiratory (Aerobic) Training

In order for your body to use stored fat to fuel muscular activities, oxygen must be present at the site of the muscle. Unlike glycogen, which is the form in which your body suspends sugars, fat cannot be broken down in the absence of oxygen. Therefore the more efficient your body becomes at taking in, transporting and delivering oxygen, the greater will be your ability to burn up any excess fat. Getting out of breath when you exercise is a sign that you are unable to provide your muscles with sufficient oxygen for them to work aerobically. When this occurs, your muscles will be relying on the breakdown of sugars (glycogen), and an organic compound called creatine phosphate, rather than using fat to supply their fuel needs. Exercising as intensely as you can, therefore, is not the best approach for fat burning. Adopting an intensity that you can sustain for an extended duration is far more effective. Walking briskly for an hour will result in far greater fat combustion than ten minutes of all-out effort.

If you are significantly overfat, avoid all high-impact activities such as jogging, running or high-impact aerobics classes, so as to protect your joints from damage. Walking, cycling, swimming, stair climbing, and some forms of dancing and rowing machines (set on a low to moderate intensity), all provide opportunities for low-impact aerobic training. Rebounding (bouncing on a mini trampoline) can be an excellent form of aerobic training and great fun as well. As you bounce, you are landing on an extremely yielding surface, so minimal stress is placed on your weight-bearing joints. It is important, however, that you maintain correct alignment of your knees as you land, as there will be a tendency for them to roll in. Making a special effort to prevent this from happening is important.

By varying the types of aerobic training you do, you can reduce any repetitive stresses on your already challenged joints. When walking, pay particular attention to your foot action. Strike the ground with your heel first and then roll through your foot before propelling yourself forward from the ball. Be cautious of walking long distances, especially in warm weather, without soft and absorbent clothing to protect your underarms and inner thighs from friction burns. Friction burns can also occur when cycling, due to your inner thighs repeatedly brushing against the seat. Padded covers are available for bicycle seats and can afford great relief from this problem.

Begin your aerobic sessions gently, at a low intensity, and then very gradually increase the degree to which you exert yourself. Remember that if you become breathless you need to reduce the intensity. If you choose to take part in an exercise-to-music class, or to follow a video with the same approach, be careful of excessive side stepping and cross steps, as they can overly challenge your vulnerable knees.

Training aerobically for 60 to 90 minutes six to seven days per week is recommended for fat loss. You may need to build up to this gradually, especially if you are severely overfat. The intensity can also be gradually progressed, such as including more hills and swinging your arms more vigorously when walking. The by-products of fat burning are carbon dioxide, water and heat. If the intensity and duration of your exercise session results in an increase in your breathing rate, the production of sweat and a feeling of warmth, then you can be assured that you are effectively burning up your stores of body fat. Not all fuel for exercise comes from your fat, since glycogen is also broken down aerobically. But although your glycogen deposits are continually replaced, you have considerably limited supplies of it at any given time. In addition, your body always keeps a little glycogen in reserve to fuel your brain and nervous system. This all means that as you perform aerobic exercise over an extended duration, your body progressively relies more on fat for its fuel source and less on glycogen.

Muscular Strength

A sluggish metabolism results in a propensity to accumulate excess body fat. While regular aerobic exercise will raise your metabolic rate for several hours following each bout of exertion, it is the development of greater muscle mass that will result in a consistently faster metabolic turnover. This is because muscle tissue has a greater metabolic demand than fat tissue. In the absence of any abnormal influences, the more muscle you have on your body the faster your metabolic rate will be 24 hours per day. This means that you will tend to process fat, and use it for fuel, far more efficiently. Consequently, you will be less likely to store it on your body. For advice on approaches to strength training, and recommended exercises, refer to Chapters Four and Five.

Muscular Endurance

The ability of your cardio-respiratory system to take in, deliver and transport oxygen becomes somewhat irrelevant if your muscles lack the ability to use the oxygen once it arrives. When you train the endurance of your muscles, you are essentially developing their efficiency to uptake oxygen. When regularly challenged by this type of training, the factories within your muscles that convert fat to fuel increase in number and size. Consequently there is a profound improvement in your ability to burn excess body fat.

General Advice for Muscular Training

If you are significantly overfat, there are a few things that you need to be aware of so as to ensure the safety and effectiveness of your muscular training. It will serve you best to focus on strengthening muscles around your weight-bearing joints (such as knees and hips) whilst not exerting any weight on them. It is recommended that you perform the following exercises six days per week, using the level of resistance that challenges you by the 18th–20th repetition:

• Seated knee extensions with ankle weights
• Seated ball squeezes for abductors
• Side lying abductor lifts
• Prone lying glute raise.

See pages 193, 126–8 and 132–3 for the relevant exercises. It is also important to exercise both the muscles and joints of your feet. Doing so will help to reduce puffiness, protect your joints, promote circulation and reduce the likelihood of varicose veins forming, and alleviate aching feet. All of these types of movements are most effective when done with bare feet. Ankle and foot exercise can be done while sitting in a chair and include the following:

• Draw clockwise and anticlockwise circles in the air with the toes (one foot at a time)
• Pick marbles up off the floor with your toes and place them in a cup (a fun game to play during TV commercials)
• Sit upright in a chair with both feet flat on the floor and raise your heels as high as you can while keeping the balls of your feet on the floor. Then place your heels back on the floor
• Sit (never do this standing) and place the outside edges of your feet on the floor, then attempt to bring the soles of your feet together by rolling your ankles outwards. Follow this by placing your feet wide apart and flat on the floor, then attempt to lift only the outsides of your feet up by rolling your ankles inwards. Throughout this exercise, pay particular attention to not push down on your thighs with your arms.

Perform as many repetitions as you feel comfortable with. The important thing is to perform these exercises with regularity.

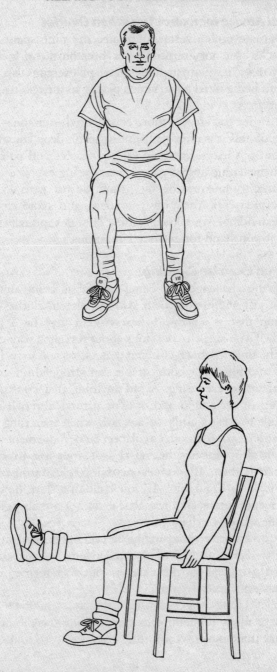

General Advice for Exercising When Overfat

If you are severely overfat, minimize the time spent lying on your back, as it can impede your breathing. Lying this way, unless you have an appropriate sized pillow, can also result in your head being tilted back, which places your neck in a vulnerable position.

The heavier you are, the more endangered your knees become. Because of this it is important not to adopt deep squatting positions that put excessive strain on your knees and patella tendons. Whenever you bend your knees, during exercise or at any other time, try to avoid bending them deeper than 45 degrees. Pay careful attention to how you stand, and avoid locking out (hyper-extending) your knee joints. This is especially likely to happen if you stand for extended durations.

A Note on Exercise Clothing

One of the challenges of being overfat is being uncomfortable, not just within your own skin but also in clothes. Finding something that is suitable to exercise in may be a problem, especially if you are self-conscious about revealing your contours. Taking the time to obtain clothing that allows you to feel psychologically and physically comfortable can strongly influence your commitment to exercising. Avoid anything that constricts your circulation or feels tight and opt for natural fibres. It is highly inadvisable to wear a girdle of any sort when exercising as it not only restricts your blood circulation and movement of your spine, but also weakens the muscles of your torso rather than strengthening them. If you feel uncomfortable in trousers, a skirt is acceptable to begin with. If you cycle in a skirt, however, be sure to secure it in such a way that it cannot possibly get entangled in the wheels or chain.

High-top exercise shoes might be preferable for you, as they offer better lateral support for your ankles. It is best to discuss your own particular footwear needs with an informed exercise-and-sports shoe salesperson.

Don't let feelings of self-consciousness rob you of the benefits of exercise. If you intend to exercise within your home, ensure that family members give you the space to do so and that they respect your privacy.

Ensure that you always have water available to drink during your exercise sessions. The more overfat you are, the more quickly you will become dehydrated. Above all, make your exercise sessions fun.

Addiction Withdrawal

The word 'addiction' is usually associated with such things as alcohol and recreational drugs, yet more people suffer from addictions to items sold as food from than any other substance. Grains, chocolate and cheese are at the top of the list when it comes to items that contain addictive substances such as opioids (opium), cannabinoids (cannabis), caffeine, theobromine, refined sugar and additives. Grains, specifically, have an impact upon your brain stem, causing it to increase its secretion of serotonin, the 'feel-good' neurotransmitter. The secretion of this natural mood enhancer automatically increases in a response to exercise. In other words if you exercised more, you would be less likely to overeat on starchy foods in order to feel comforted and happier.

Fresh raw fruits and vegetables do not contain any addictive substances. For this reason you never hear of people being 'addicted' to peaches, oranges, lettuce or broccoli! There is only one way to get free of an addiction and that is to go through the discomfort of withdrawal. It seldom works to wean yourself off a substance that you have become addicted to. If you are uncertain what your food addictions may be, for a couple of days eat only fresh fruits and vegetables and then gradually reintroduce other items one at a time. Any food that you find yourself obsessing about, or eating compulsively, is a food to which you are addicted. If you suffer from any specific health problems, however, check with your doctor before experimenting with your diet in this way.

As you pass through the challenge of withdrawal from your addictions, the thing that can help you most is exercise. Physical exertion releases pent up stress, stimulates your own production of serotonin, provides you with time out from the pressure of life, and leaves you with a feeling of well being.

Emotional Independence from Food

This is probably the most challenging of the ingredients for a healthy body weight. Comfort eating is not just a theory; it is a

fact. Every time you eat, your body has to expend energy processing the food. The more you eat and the greater the digestive challenge, the less energy you have available to conduct emotions.

There are only two healthy reasons for eating: nourishment and
pleasure. Although it is common for overeaters to believe that
their over indulgences result from an excessive pursuit of pleasure
(greed), the truth is that the root causes of overeating are emotional discomfort and addiction. The healthiest way to cope with
emotional distress is to take the time to actually feel it. This
involves stepping off the merry-go-round of everyday frenetic
living, sitting alone somewhere quiet and allowing your emotions
to surface. Depending on your personal history and psychological
disposition, this might be best done under the guidance of a
trained counsellor. Moving into the second half of your life is the
perfect time to free yourself from the burdens of accumulated
emotional baggage and set yourself free to enjoy the pleasures of
being a wiser and more relaxed person.

Osteoporosis

Calcium and phosphorous are constantly being released from
your bones. This is because they are needed elsewhere in your
body for such things as muscular activity and neural functioning.
These minerals are also regularly replaced so that the integrity of
your bones is maintained. An additional and very important role
of calcium is its use as an alkaline buffer should the pH of your
blood become disturbed by excessive acidity. Your blood needs to
be maintained at 7.40 (slightly alkaline) and any significant deviation from this can result in death. Due to the poor dietary and
lifestyle habits of most people in the Western world, their blood
pH is constantly becoming too acid. This results in vast amounts
of calcium being regularly leached from their bones as the body
tries to negate the excess acidity and return the blood to its pre-
dominately alkaline state. This de-mineralization of the bone
tissue causes it to lose its density and strength.

The outer layer of your bones is referred to as compact or cor-
tical bone. It is very dense and, in healthy bones, extremely strong.
The inner portion is comprised of a honeycomb structure,
referred to as cancellous or spongy bone. When your bones lose
their mineral content faster than it is replaced, the cancellous bone

gradually disintegrates, its honeycomb structure breaking down into a series of gaping holes. The compact bone suffers too, shrinking in diameter and losing its strength. The result is that your bones become highly vulnerable to fracturing. Once in this diseased state, it may only take a bumpy car ride for you to break your ribs or a trip on the pavement for you to fracture a hip.

Body Area at High Risk from Fracturing
• Ankles
• Hips
• Lumbar spine
• Thoracic spine
• Cervical spine
• Shoulders
• Radius (wrist)

Note: Hand laundering large items provides excellent strengthening for the muscles of your forearms.

Signs and Symptoms of Osteoporosis
Although backache can occur for a variety of reasons, persistent lower back pain is often the first indication of osteoporosis. Other symptoms include pain elsewhere in the body, inhibited ranges of motion and visually identifiable malformations such as a stooped posture (hyperkyphosis). Diagnosis is possible in the form of X-rays or bone scans. Often, it is only when a person presents a fracture for medical attention that osteoporosis is tested for and diagnosed.

Osteoporosis is not a natural part of the ageing process. Instead it is caused by the accumulation of acid forming dietary and lifestyle habits coupled with long-term inactivity.

Exercise Guidelines for Bone Strengthening
The same applies here as for all the conditions mentioned in this chapter so far: because a lack of exercise is not the sole cause of the condition, addressing it alone while ignoring the other factors will not bring about healing. In order to prevent osteoporosis, or to heal from it, you need to incorporate the information from Chapter One into your plan, as well as applying the following exercise recommendations.

The two types of activity that most effectively stimulate the bones to stay strong are those involving skeletal impact and those requiring muscular strength.

Muscular Strength

Exercises requiring muscular strength place stresses on your bones as a result of the muscles pulling on them via the tendons. Of special value are exercises that strengthen the muscles surrounding sites at high risk from fracturing. This is because stronger muscles provide these areas with better support and strengthen the bones specifically in those vulnerable areas.

Strengthening muscles that improve your physical poise and posture are also vital if spinal deformity is to be avoided and your risk of falling minimized. Here is a list of the recommended muscle groups to strengthen, in accordance with the areas of your body that are most vulnerable to fracturing as a result of osteoporosis. Turn to Chapter Five for the appropriate exercises.

Body Area at High Risk from Fracturing	Muscles to Strengthen
Ankles	Fronts and backs of calves
Hips	Insides and outsides of thighs and buttocks
Lumbar spine	Abdominals and lower back muscles
Thoracic spine	Upper back muscles
Cervical spine	Neck muscles
Shoulders	Front, back and top of shoulders
Radius (wrist)	Forearms muscles

NB: Hand laundering large items provides excellent strengthening for the muscles of your forearms.

Skeletal Impact

The word 'impact' is used to describe the force with which one object collides with another. Within the context of exercise, the word is used when referring to the degree of trauma that the feet are exposed to as they strike the ground. When an exercise is said to be high impact, it is usually because it includes jumping upwards, from one or both feet, followed by a correspondingly forceful landing. Not all high impact is preceded by jumping; stamping of the feet when marching, for example, applies considerable force to the feet. Impact produces shock waves that travel directly along the line of trauma until they are dispersed, absorbed or dissipated. It is these shock waves that can trigger bone anabolism (bone building), resulting in stronger bones.

In a similar way that muscular strength can be developed by the use of resistance work, bone strength can be improved via the challenge of impact. In addition to improving the quality of your bone mass, skeletal impact work can also develop your leg power and balance, as well as the speed and efficiency of your neuromuscular pathways (the pathways of communication between your brain and muscles).

The degree of impact must be appropriate to the condition of your bones and, importantly, the health of your joints. If you suffer from arthritis to any significant degree, even moderate impact will be inappropriate for you. If this is the case, focus more on strength training, as described above. Another factor that will render impact work inappropriate is advanced osteoporosis, as it places you at risk from fractures should you attempt this form of exercise. If you are in any doubt whatsoever, it is vital that you consult with your health care professional before beginning a programme of skeletal impact.

NB: Do not attempt this type of exercise if any of the following conditions apply to you:

- Arthritis
- Significant osteoporosis
- Obesity
- Soft tissue acute injuries or other inflammation
- Acute infections
- Parkinson's disease
- Recent invasive medical treatment, e.g. surgery
- Recent concussion (common as a result of falling)
- Excessively poor posture
- Vertigo or other balance problems
- Stroke-induced hyper/hypo muscle tone
- Disorders of the retina

- Incontinence
- Hip or knee replacements
- Whiplash
- Ulcerated varicose veins
- Colostomy
- Severe distortions of the feet.

Provided that none of the above applies to you, it is safe for you to perform bone-loading exercises. In order to transmit some shock waves through your skeletal system to stimulate the bone-building cells, the following exercises can be done:

Lower Body Bone-loading Exercises (up to and Including the Lower Back)

Walking
This needs to be done in a dynamic manner, preferably uphill and downhill. Providing your lower back, hips, knees, and ankle joints are free from arthritis, it is more effective to wear thinner, rather than thicker, soled shoes for the purpose of bone loading.

Jogging or Running
This is only suitable for you when osteoporosis is a *risk,* and unsuitable if your bones are *already* osteoporotic. Once again, if you are unsure, consult your health care professional.

Springing
This exercise will stimulate bone-building cells throughout your legs, pelvis and lower spine.

Starting position: Standing with the feet parallel and at about hip-distance apart, bend the knees slightly without allowing the upper body to tip forwards.

Movement: Propel yourself upwards into a shallow spring (just high enough so that a sheet of paper could slide between your feet and the floor). As you land, be sure to bend the knees and bring the heels all the way down to the floor. Repeat the exercise 20 times three times each day. Perform the exercise with either bare feet or shoes with no heels such as trainers.

Essential technique:

- Warm up properly before performing springing by thoroughly mobilising your ankles, knees and hips (see Chapter Four). Bend by flexing your knees and ankles prior to springing. Be sure your knees are kept in line over your toes
- Avoid excessive flexion at your hips, which will result in tipping you forwards
- Lengthen your body upwards during the elevation phase
- Keep your shoulders above your hips on both take off and landing. In other words, do not allow your torso to twist
- Land with your weight equally distributed over *both* feet
- Land through your feet with a ball-to-heel motion
- Bend your ankles and knees as your feet make contact with the floor on landing
- Control the landing by keeping your knees in line over your toes and your abdominal muscles tight
- Only straighten your legs on landing once your heels are down and you have regained your balance.

Upper Body Bone-loading Exercises

Hand Clapping (Wrists)
This is the simplest exercise in this book. Clap your hands together at least 100 times a day to strengthen the bones in your wrists. This activity does not need to be done all in one go. Seek out opportunities to offer applause. Not only will you strengthen your bones, but you will also become appreciated for your recognition of other people's efforts!

Wall drops (Wrists and Shoulders)
Starting position: Stand slightly further than arms length away from a wall with your arms extended out in front of you at shoulder height. Your palms should be facing the wall with fingers pointing towards the ceiling. Place the feet parallel to each other and at about hip-distance apart.

Movement: Pulling in your abdominal muscles so that your back does not 'sway', drop forwards onto the wall and catch yourself on your hands. Your heels will rise slightly off the floor as you do so. Maintaining tight abdominal muscles and a straight back, push yourself back up to an upright position. Repeat the movement 20 times, breathing naturally as you do so. As your arms get stronger and your abdominal strength improves, you will gradually be able to stand further away from the wall.

Seated Drops (Entire Spine)

Starting position: Sit in a hard chair with both feet flat on the floor and about hip-width apart. Ensure that your knees are over your ankles and that you are sitting upright with good posture. Grasp each side of the chair's seat with your hands, tilting slightly forwards from the hips as you do so. Push down with your hands and feet, as if you were going to stand up, until you have raised your bottom so that it *just* loses contact with the chair seat. Then let yourself drop heavily back down onto the chair. Perform 4 to 6 repetitions of the seated drops, and then take a break before repeating them. Aim to perform four sets of 4 to 6 repetitions each day.

Essential technique:

• Ensure that you lengthen your neck throughout the exercise and look straight ahead.

A Note on Swimming and Cycling

Due to the non-weight-bearing nature of swimming and cycling, they are of minimal benefit in terms of providing the necessary shock waves to stimulate osteoblasts activity. However, because of the muscular work involved in these activities, the pulling of the muscles on the bones is effective in helping to keep the bones strong. Swimming and cycling are also useful for strengthening muscles around areas at high risk from fracturing.

Chapter 7
Choosing Your Fun and Where to Find It

The greatest influence upon whether or not you adhere to your fitness regimen, and achieve your goals, is how much you look forward to and enjoy your exercise sessions. A programme of exercise that is perfectly designed to meet your physical needs is of minimal value to you if your motivation wanes and your practice of it dissolves. It is far better to choose activities that may be marginally less effective, but which you adhere to for years to come and delight in every moment spent pursuing them, than to allow the 'perfect' type of exercise to become a drudgery that you quickly discontinue.

Variety is not just the spice of life; it is also the spice of exercising. Rather than limiting yourself to one or two approaches to fitness training, consider exploring a variety of activities. What follows is a selection of different approaches that you can take to training the five different components of fitness. It is not fully inclusive and there are many other sports, games, recreational activities, pastimes, fitness pursuits and hobbies that you can try out. The exciting news is that the fitter you are the greater variety of fun activities you can enjoy. Beware of declaring that you do not enjoy something if you have never tried it, or you may miss out on some delightful fitness enhancing opportunities.

The activities are listed in alphabetical order for ease of reference. The form of fitness training relevant to each activity is also explained. In Appendix 2 you will find listed contact details for where you can find further information.

Aquarobics
Description: A water-based exercise class, sometimes accompanied by music, whereby the resistance and buoyancy provided by the water is used to develop various aspects of fitness.

For Training Aerobic Fitness: A well-designed class can provide very effective training for your cardio-respiratory system.

For Developing Muscular Strength: Although the emphasis tends to be on endurance, the resistance of the water does provide opportunities for some development of strength. The degree to which this type of training is included depends on each individual aquarobics teacher. If you have significant arthritis of your hands, high blood pressure or angina, or suffer from transient ischaemic attacks (ITAs), then avoid strength work altogether and focus instead on developing muscular endurance.

For Developing Muscular Endurance: An excellent method of developing a comprehensive (whole body) range of endurance.

For Increasing/Maintaining Flexibility: Due to the support provided by the water, some ranges of movement can be more confidently developed than when attempted on dry land.

For Training of Motor Fitness: Your coordination and reaction time are exercised as you follow the teacher's instructions. Aquarobics provides you with an excellent opportunity to practise developing your balance, as if you fall there is virtually no risk of injury.

Equipment and Gear Needed: A swimsuit. Some establishments request that you wear a swimming cap, although this is very rarely the case with aquarobics, as you are not asked to submerge your head under the water.

Advantages: Classes are taken in the shallow end of a swimming pool, with a water level of about chest height. If you are a non-swimmer you can, therefore, partake with confidence. The virtual absence of skeletal impact is one of the greatest advantages of water-based exercise, as it means that you can achieve vigorous aerobic training with minimal stress to your bones and joints. This is an obvious advantage if you suffer from arthritis or other joint problems, or are significantly overweight. Another advantage of the buoyancy and support provided by the water is that it allows for the exploration and maintenance of greater ranges of movement than you might feel confident to achieve on dry land. Due to the high humidity, all water-based activities are helpful if you suffer from breathing difficulties such as asthma. Aquarobics classes are usually fun and allow for plenty of social interaction, and are a good way to become confident in water if you are a non-swimmer.

Disadvantages: Due to the lack of skeletal impact, water-based exercise is not helpful in stimulating the bone-building cells needed for the healing of osteoporosis. If muscular strength work is included, however, osteoblasts can be stimulated in this way. The chemicals present in the water of public facilities are toxic and unhealthful. The distance between the nearest class and your home may be considerable and therefore getting there may be a problem for you. The surfaces around a swimming pool can be slippery, so be sure to take special care not to fall.

Unsuitable: If you are self-conscious about being seen in a swimming costume, have an open wound, difficulty in hearing or suffer from uncontrolled epilepsy.

Opportunity: Most sports and leisure centres that have swimming pools offer aquarobics classes. Once you have learnt the techniques involved it is possible for you to practice on your own at the shallow end of your local pool.

Cost: Classes typically cost between £3 and £5.

Badminton

Description: A racket sport, using a shuttlecock, played by two or four players.

For Training Aerobic Fitness: Badminton is generally a start-and-stop type of sport. If you are a beginner, you will spend more time walking over to pick your shuttlecock up off the floor than you will actually hitting it with your racket. Once you become an experienced player each bout of exertion is short-lived, with a pause in between. Badminton is therefore not especially effective for developing your aerobic fitness, as it is more of an anaerobic challenge.

For Developing Muscular Strength: A comprehensive range of strength is required for badminton, specifically of the arms and shoulders. Leg strength can also be challenged by this game once a moderate level of play is achieved. The more skilled a player you become, the more overall strength you will require.

For Developing Muscular Endurance: As the game consists of short bursts of explosive exertion, followed by a pause, it is not typically effective at developing endurance. However, badminton can provide endurance training for a very comprehensive range of muscles, if the goal of play is to sustain a volley of continual movement.

<u>For Increasing/Maintaining Flexibility</u>: Flexibility of the shoulders, inner thighs, back, and sides of the torso are needed to play badminton.

<u>For Training of Motor Fitness</u>: A superb way to train your reaction times and speed. Your coordination is also developed and some degree of balance is required.

<u>Equipment and Gear Needed</u>: If you play at a sports or leisure centre, they may well be able to hire out a racket and shuttle-cocks; otherwise you will need to purchase these items. Trainers specifically designed for the game are necessary if you become a regular player. When first trying out the game, a pair of cross-trainers (general-purpose sports shoes) will suffice.

<u>Advantages</u>: All racket sports potentially provide opportunities for social interaction. They are also excellent for stimulating the bone-building cells via skeletal trauma. Shock waves resulting from the ball meeting the racket travel up the wrist, arm and shoulder – a great asset if osteoporosis is a concern for you.

<u>Disadvantages</u>: Your play is restricted by the accessibility of a court and availability of a partner.

<u>Unsuitable</u>: If you have high blood pressure or angina, or suffer from transient ischaemic attacks (ITAs), arthritis (especially of the shoulders, neck or hands), whiplash injury, lower back pain, Parkinson's disease, frozen shoulder, fibromyalgia, vertigo or severe kyphosis (stooped posture).

<u>Opportunity</u>: Almost all leisure and sports centres provide badminton courts.

<u>Cost</u>: The use of a court varies quite a bit, but is usually between £5 and £10 per hour.

Bowls

<u>Description</u>: This game can be played indoors or outdoors. It involves rolling heavy balls along the ground in an attempt to get them as close as possible to a target ball that is placed some distance away.

<u>For Training Aerobic Fitness</u>: None to any significant degree.

<u>For Developing Muscular Strength</u>: Develops strength of the arm and shoulder of your playing arm. In order to have equal

strength on your non-playing side, you need either to train that arm or shoulder separately or become an ambidextrous bowler! If you have weak thigh muscles, playing bowls can develop some strength in this area.

For Developing Muscular Endurance: None to any significant degree.

For Increasing/Maintaining Flexibility: This game only requires flexibility of your playing shoulder and a small degree of flexibility in your lower back and hips.

For Training of Motor Fitness: Spatial awareness and depth perception are key to playing bowls. Some degree of balance and coordination is also needed.

Equipment and Gear Needed: None except for the bowling balls and a surface upon which to play.

Advantages: A gentle and sociable game that can provide a starting point for you, if your fitness is very poor.

Disadvantages: Overall, playing bowls provides minimal fitness gains.

Unsuitable: If you have significant arthritis of your knees, neck or hands. Bowls is also unsuitable if you have a frozen shoulder (of your playing arm), suffer from lower back pain, have severe sight problems, severe kyphosis or whiplash injury.

Opportunity: Most leisure and sports centres provide the opportunity to play bowls, many of which run clubs. There are also many independent locally run bowling clubs.

Cost: Typically between £2.50 and £3.50 per person plus membership if you join a club.

Callisthenics

Description: Specific exercises, predominantly floor-based, whereby you use your own body and gravity in order to develop muscular strength and endurance.

For Training Aerobic Fitness: None of any significance.

For Developing Muscular Strength: The degree to which any given callisthenic exercise can train the strength or endurance of your muscles depends upon the design of the exercise and your current level of strength. If you have high blood pressure or angina, or suffer from transient ischaemic attacks (ITAs), then avoid strength work altogether until you have resolved the problem by removing the causes (see Chapters One and Two). Until that time, focus instead on developing muscular endurance. In the case of Parkinson's disease, strength training is best avoided. Light endurance work, accompanied by an extensive amount of stretching, is recommended instead.

For Developing Muscular Endurance: See above.

For Increasing/Maintaining Flexibility: If callisthenics are executed utilizing your full potential of movement ranges, then it is a way to maintain your flexibility. Performing callisthenics will not increase or develop your flexibility.

For Training of Motor Fitness: Balance is required for some callisthenic exercises, and performing them with correct technique depends upon body awareness and coordination.

Equipment and Gear Needed: Non-restrictive clothing and an exercise mat.

Advantages: A comprehensive training of all your major muscle groups can be achieved through a well-constructed programme of callisthenics. It is inappropriate for resistance machines, bands, free weights or other external forms of resistance to be used until you have the strength to perform basic callisthenics managing your own body weight. Providing you learn, and practise correct exercise technique, this is an excellent way to improve your body awareness and posture.

Disadvantages: Unless you are very experienced, or practise under the watchful eye of a fitness teacher, you are likely to perform the exercises with poor technique, resulting in reduced effectiveness and possible injury.

Unsuitable: Many callisthenic exercises may be unsuitable for you if you are unable to get down onto the floor or have significant arthritis of the knees or hips. With the help of an experienced fitness teacher you can learn to adapt most exercises by performing them in positions where you are sitting or standing. Many callisthenic exercises will also need adapting for you if you have severe kyphosis or a frozen shoulder. If you have Parkinson's disease, you are better to work on stretching and low-intensity rhythmical movements. Avoid all intensities that challenge your strength if you suffer from this disease.

Opportunity: Once you have learnt the exercises and correct techniques, either by attending a class or working with a personal trainer, you can perform callisthenic exercises safely and effectively at home.

Cost: Classes run at leisure and sports centres typically cost between £3 and £5. Such sessions are often referred to as body sculpting classes, or toning classes, or are given catchy names. If you opt for a personal trainer, the cost can vary enormously; your local fitness centre will be able to advise you.

Circuit Training

Description: An instructor-led group session whereby individuals, partners or small sub-groups rotate around a series of pre-set exercise stations. The stations typically consist of resistance equipment, callisthenic exercises (see above) or a mixture of both.

For Training Aerobic Fitness: Although some circuits are designed exclusively to train aerobic fitness, this is rare. More commonly muscular strength and endurance training is the goal.

For Developing Muscular Strength: This depends entirely on the design of the circuit and your current level of strength. Typically, there will be a predominance of endurance work with the addition of a few stations that challenge your strength. If you have high blood pressure or angina or suffer from transient ischaemic attacks (ITAs), then avoid strength work altogether until you have resolved the problem by removing the causes (see Chapters One and Two). Until that time, focus instead on developing muscular endurance. In the case of Parkinson's disease, strength training is best avoided. Light endurance work, accompanied by an extensive amount of stretching, is recommended.

For Developing Muscular Endurance: See directly above.

For Increasing/Maintaining Flexibility: A well-designed and safely taught circuit training session will always finish with a comprehensive stretching out of all the muscles that you have been working. This will help you to maintain your current ranges of movement. It is unusual for circuit training classes to include significant time increasing and developing flexibility.

For Training of Motor Fitness: A well-designed circuit will require some degree of motor fitness training, although this will be incidental rather than a primary goal.

Equipment and Gear Needed: Non-restrictive clothing that allows your bodyline to be viewed by the instructor.

Advantages: Due to the team approach, this form of exercise can be highly motivating.

Disadvantages: If you are a beginner, or lack confidence, you may find the sometimes dictatorial and hyper-dynamic approach adopted by some teachers rather intimidating. Circuit training tends to bring out the competitive side of people, which can result in attempts to achieve more than is appropriate.

Unsuitable: This depends to a very large degree on the type of circuit you participate in. If it is a floor-based class, then the same applies as for callisthenics (see above). Due to the tendency for people to compete and the typically fast and intense pace of circuit training, it is an unsuitable form of exercise if you have high blood pressure or angina, or other heart-related health problems. If you have had a hip replacement, moderate to severe kyphosis, or whiplash injury, be sure to check with the instructor beforehand whether the class will be suitable for you. Circuit training is not recommended if you have hearing problems. This is because such sessions usually take place in large echoing sports halls, and there is typically a great deal of noise as people chat while exercising.

Opportunity: Most sports and leisure centres run circuit training classes. Once you have been to a few classes to gather ideas and learn correct exercise technique, it may be possible for you to set up your own circuit stations at home if that suits you better than attending group sessions.

Cost: Costs vary but are typically around £3.50 per session.

Cardio-Gym

Description: A room filled with a variety of machines designed to challenge your aerobic fitness such as treadmills, stair climbers and stationary bicycles. Also referred to as walking/jogging/running machines, treadmills provide the opportunity for imitating the mechanics of these activities while remaining indoors.

For Training Aerobic Fitness: Specifically designed for this purpose and very effective.

For Developing Muscular Strength: If you have set the intensity of what you are attempting so high as to challenge your strength, you will not be training your cardio-respiratory system.

For Developing Muscular Endurance: Every machine will exercise at least one aspect of your muscular endurance.

<u>For Increasing/Maintaining Flexibility</u>: Not effective.

<u>For Training of Motor Fitness</u>: Some coordination may be required for some machines, but generally this approach to training will not develop your motor skills.

<u>Equipment and Gear Needed</u>: Non-restrictive clothing that can be removed in layers as you get warmer. A pair of appropriate exercise shoes such as cross-trainers.

<u>Advantages</u>: Most machines provide high-tech, accurate figures on the duration, intensity and progress of your training. On many machines you can pre-set your workout intensity and duration. As it is done indoors, cardio-gym is a good option if you are a fair weather exerciser or have fears for your personal safety when outside. This form of training also provides an opportunity to train aerobically if after dark is your only available time to do so. The advantage of treadmills is that the machines can be set at a speed to suit your needs, and most have elaborate technology enabling you to evaluate such things as the distance you have covered, the number of calories you have expended and your average speed. The surface of a treadmill provides a much softer foot strike than walking or jogging on the road. This is of especial value if you have arthritis. The intensity of the challenge can be altered to suit your training programme, by increasing or decreasing the speed of the machine. If you like to walk, jog or run but dislike doing so in wet weather, then a treadmill may be an answer for you.

<u>Disadvantages</u>: Training with machines can be uninspiring and, unless you are technologically minded, you might find the array of dials, displays and buttons intimidating. Exercising indoors, instead of obtaining the fresh air and natural sunlight that accompanies outdoor aerobic-based pursuits, cannot generally be considered the healthy option. Exercising on a treadmill can be boring and monotonous. It is possible to fall off a treadmill, especially if your balance is not reasonably well developed. Unless you invest in your own treadmill, you are restricted to exercising within the times available at the gym. Travelling to the gym may be a problem for you.

<u>Unsuitable</u>: The use of this type of equipment is not recommended if you suffer from vertigo. If you have an attack, you may be unable to get off the machine and may fall, or get into

other difficulties. Treadmills are specifically unsuitable if you have:

- Arthritis of the feet, knees, hips, hands or neck
- Vertigo or other balance problems
- Sight problems
- Hearing problems (because your balance may be affected)
- Epilepsy
- Parkinson's disease.

NB: It is important that a qualified fitness instructor shows you how to use the machines safely and effectively. It is especially important to learn how to get on and off them safely. This is exceptionally important if you have a hip replacement, significant osteoporosis or suffer from Parkinson's disease.

Opportunity: Most leisure centres, sports centres and fitness clubs have CV machinery. You can buy your own, but they take up a great deal of space.

Cost: The use of CV machinery varies greatly. Private clubs can be expensive but your local leisure or sports centre will probably charge between £3 and £5 per session. Buying you own equipment is very expensive.

The cost of a treadmill varies between about £2,000 and £3,500, mainly depending on the extent of technological gadgetry provided. For details on where to obtain a treadmill, refer to the resources section at the back of the book.

Cricket

Description: A team sport played out of doors on a green, using a bat, a hard ball and small vertical posts pushed into the ground.

For Training Aerobic Fitness: Bouts of exertion are short-lived with long pauses in between, making cricket an ineffective way to develop aerobic fitness.

For Developing Muscular Strength: This depends upon your position of play. Only when you bat or throw the ball is strength required in your arms and shoulders. Overall, cricket is ineffective in training your body's strength.

For Developing Muscular Endurance: Some degree of lower body endurance is required when your position is that of fielder.

For Increasing/Maintaining Flexibility: Flexibility of your shoulders is required to play cricket, and the frequent bending down to pick the ball up from the ground provides a good opportunity to maintain functional flexibility of your hips, knees and lower back.

For Training of Motor Fitness: This game demands eye-to-hand coordination, fast reaction times and some degree of agility.

Equipment and Gear Needed: Very specific to the sport and your position of play. Your cricket club will be able to advise you.

Advantages: Cricket provides an opportunity for social interaction and team play. The degree of overall exertion is generally low, but this depends upon the standard of the team with whom you are playing, and is governed by your own level of fitness.

Disadvantages: Practice and matches may only take place once a week or less. If you join a club as a beginner, the amount of actual physical activity you experience may be minimal.

Unsuitable: If you have severe arthritis anywhere in your body, a frozen shoulder, lower back pain (as there is a lot of standing and a considerable amount of bending involved), or severe kyphosis.

Opportunity: This may be a problem when travelling, or on holiday, as you will typically be restricted to playing exclusively with your local team.

Cost: Varies from county to county.

Cycling

Description: Riding a bicycle, tricycle or tandem either on the road or off-road, depending on what it is designed for and your preference.

For Training Aerobic Fitness: Cycling is a potentially excellent and effective way to develop your aerobic fitness.

For Developing Muscular Strength: Strength of your legs and arms is needed for cycling up steep inclines. This type of cycling is not recommended if you have high blood pressure or angina, or suffer from transient ischaemic attacks (ITAs).

For Developing Muscular Endurance: Cycling is especially effective for developing the endurance of your leg muscles.

For Increasing/Maintaining Flexibility: Not effective.

For Training of Motor Fitness: With the exception of riding a tricycle, a highly tuned ability to balance is required for cycling.

A quick reaction time is also needed for safe cycling and coordination is challenged to some degree.

Equipment and Gear Needed: A bicycle. If you are trying out this activity, there is no need to purchase your own as there are many shops that hire bicycles of all descriptions and sizes. A safety helmet is recommended and is a necessity if you intend to ride on the roads. Cycling shorts provide extra padding for your sitting bones and protect your inner thighs from chaffing. Gloves are recommended and are a great asset if you intend to ride off-road, in cold weather or are prone to blisters. Gloves also help to protect your hands should you fall. Unless you are an advanced rider who undertakes competitive cycling, a well fitting pair of trainers provides adequate footwear. What you wear on the rest of your body depends upon your level of fitness, the type of cycling you intend to do and the weather conditions. Dressing in layers is preferable and this means that you will need panniers on your bicycle, or a backpack, in order to have somewhere to put clothes as you warm up and strip off.

Advantages: Cycling can be great fun and a sociable activity that all age groups can enjoy together. It provides a highly effective form of aerobic and endurance training and can be used as an alternative method of transport; saving money, the environment, and your health.

Disadvantages: You might live in a location where heavy traffic renders cycling an undesirable pastime.

Unsuitable: If you suffer from severe arthritis in your hands, have arthritis to any significant degree in your neck, or have a whiplash injury, then cycling is not the best option for you. If you suffer from osteoporosis, you are better off relying on weight-bearing activities such as walking for developing your aerobic fitness. Cycling is not suitable for you if you suffer from vertigo, or have other balance problems. Cycling can exacerbate lower back pain, although altering the height of the seat in relation to the handlebars can sometimes alleviate this. Significant problems with sight would make cycling dangerous, as would uncontrolled epilepsy. Avoid cycling off-road or on uneven ground if you have a detached/partially detached retina. If you have severe kyphosis, then cycling is not the activity for you.

<u>Opportunity</u>: With the exception of traffic problems, cycling can be done almost anywhere. If you are in the country, following the bridleways will ensure you have no gates or styles to lift your bicycle over. Remember, cycling on footpaths is not allowed, so if you use them you need to be prepared to get off and push! Cycling clubs exist all over the country and many accommodate weekend leisure seekers as well as seriously competitive athletes.

<u>Cost</u>: If you decide to cycle regularly then you will need to purchase your own bicycle. Prices range from around £200 to well over £2,000 and beyond. Bicycles fall into essentially three design categories: those designed for riding exclusively on an even surface such as a road or purpose-built competitive cycling track; those designed for off-road cycling over uneven ground and mountainous terrain; and those that will accommodate both types of riding to a compromised and modest degree. The cost of a helmet, and any other accessories that you deem necessary, varies greatly according to quality. Once you have purchased these items, the ongoing cost of cycling is very small. You can, of course, pay to join a cycling club, which you would need to consider within your budget.

Dancing

<u>Description</u>: Any form of creative physical movement that is either choreographed or spontaneous. Dance is typically performed in rhythm with music, but music is not always used. Here we will look at ballet and ballroom dancing, ballet because it has so much to offer from a fitness perspective and ballroom dancing because it typically appeals to older adults.

Ballet is a specific type of tightly structured classical dance with an emphasis on correct technique, reaching maximal ranges of movement, and optimal physical elegance. You do not need to be young, nor slim, nor female, to enjoy and reap the enormous benefits of ballet.

Ballroom dancing is a type of choreographed dance requiring partners, the origins of which date back some centuries, performed to classical instrumental music.

<u>Training Specifics</u>: There is such a wide variety of movement types that can be classified as dance that it is impossible to give a generalized rating for effectiveness in training the five different

components of fitness. A lot also depends on your standard of expertise and performance. The type of dance you do depends on your physical condition and your preferences. Without exception, however, all forms of dance will train your balance and coordination, as well as develop your body awareness.

For Training Aerobic Fitness: Ballet – the more skilled you become at ballet, the more you will be able to develop your aerobic fitness through completing dance patterns of an extended duration. As a beginner, much of your time will be spent learning the steps and techniques.

Ballroom dancing – the degree to which ballroom dancing challenges your aerobic fitness depends upon how fit your cardio-respiratory system is, and how skilled and dynamic your dancing is. Certainly it will provide an excellent degree of exertion for you if you are a beginner who is less fit.

For Developing Muscular Strength: Ballet – this is a highly effective way to develop the strength of your lower body. Upper body strength is not significantly challenged, with the exception of male dancers of an advanced level who lift their female partners.

Ballroom dancing – your strength will not be challenged by this form of exercise.

For Developing Muscular Endurance: Ballet – this is one of the most effective ways to develop endurance in all of your body's skeletal muscles.

Ballroom dancing – due to its continuous and rhythmical nature, ballroom dancing will provide excellent training for the endurance of your leg muscles. The muscles of your shoulders will develop some stamina too, as you will hold your arms in a poised position with your partner's.

For Increasing/Maintaining Flexibility: Ballet – a very effective way to develop a comprehensive range of flexibility throughout your arms, torso, and legs.

Ballroom dancing – the longer and wider strides involved in some dances will go a long way to help you to maintain flexibility of your thighs and the muscles surrounding your hips.

For Training of Motor Fitness: Balance, reaction time and coordination are all extensively developed by ballet and, to a lesser degree, by ballroom dancing.

Equipment and Gear Needed: This varies tremendously according to the type of dance that you participate in, especially with regard to footwear. Your teacher will be able to advise you.

Ballet – clothing that allows for unrestricted movement and enables your bodyline to be clearly visible to your teacher. Ballet shoes.

Ballroom dancing – requires clothing that is non-restrictive and preferably shoes specifically designed for this type of dance. If you are a beginner, a pair of well-fitting shoes that are not likely to slip on a wooden floor, nor have thick treads, are acceptable.

Advantages: The creative expression of the dance can easily become the focal point rather than the 'exercising just to get fit' approach. This means that it is more likely to be something you develop a passion for and look forward to on each occasion, resulting in long-term adherence. Unlike other more regimented approaches to movement, dance encourages your body's own naturally unique way of moving to develop.

Ballet – one of the very best forms of exercise for you to develop greater body awareness and improve your posture. Ballroom dancing – a very sociable and fun way to exercise. The intensity of exertion can be adapted to suit your fitness level.

Disadvantages: Some types of dance require that you have a partner, although this is rarely a problem as people pair up in classes. You may find a need to augment your dancing with other forms of exercise due to the fact that your dance class is only held once a week. There may be time spent standing around while others, who do not learn the steps as quickly as you do, get individual help.

Ballet – men may view ballet as an essentially feminine form of movement, but this is purely a perception. Ballet has vast fitness benefits for both men and women.

Ballroom dancing – finding a partner who is willing to dance with you on a regular basis is ideal, but is not always easy. Most classes will find you a partner if you do not have one, but they may not be of your standard.

Unsuitable: With the exception of some forms of paralysis, there is no condition for which dance cannot be rendered suitable.

Ballet – unsuitable if you have arthritis of your hips, knees or feet. Ballet is also unsuitable if you have severe osteoporosis, have had a hip replacement, have severe kyphosis, a detached/partially detached retina, or bunions.

Ballroom dancing – unsuitable if you have severe arthritis of the feet or hips, or painful bunions.

Opportunity: Classes are run by leisure centres, adult education programmes, dance schools, and independent teachers. Your local dancewear shop should be able to put you in touch with teachers in your area.

Ballet – classes for children are to be found in even the smallest of villages. It can be difficult, however, to find classes for adult beginners.

Ballroom dancing – classes may be a little difficult to track down. Your local adult education centre is a good place to start. Once you have learnt the basics, you can practise with your partner at home and display your talents at social gatherings.

Cost: The cost of classes varies considerably from class to class and area to area.

Ballet – usually between £3.50 and £7 per class, depending on the length of the class and the geographical area. Private lessons are sometimes available and cost more accordingly.

Ballroom dancing – usually between £3.50 and £7 per class, depending on the length of the class and the geographical area. Private lessons are sometimes available and cost more accordingly. There is usually a discount for couples.

Exercise to Music

Description: A class where exercises are performed to the beat, phrase and rhythm of music. Classes typically consist of a warm-up, an aerobic training component, callisthenics to develop muscular strength and endurance and a cool-down stretch. The amount of time spent on each part of the class varies according to individual teachers and the level of fitness the class is intended for.

For Training Aerobic Fitness: Fun and very effective. The aerobic section of the class is based on a dance-like approach. It may be all low-impact, or a mixture of low- (one foot is always in contact with the floor) and high-impact (both feet momentarily leaving the ground) moves. A well-designed class does not consist of exclusively high-impact steps.

For Developing Muscular Strength: If you are a beginner, some of the callisthenic exercises (see page 207) will challenge your strength. Once you reach an intermediate level, there is typically very little that will train this aspect of your fitness.

For Developing Muscular Endurance: Highly effective and comprehensive.

For Increasing/Maintaining Flexibility: A well-designed class will devote significant time, towards the end, for the development of your flexibility.

For Training of Motor Fitness: The complexity of the aerobic dance will be gauged according to the level of the class (beginners, intermediate or advanced). Balance, coordination, agility and reaction time are all trained very effectively in an ETM class.

Equipment and Gear Needed: A pair of fitness shoes specifically designed for these types of classes, with extra cushioning under the balls of your feet. Non-restrictive clothing that allows your bodyline to be seen and that can be removed in layers as you get warmer.

Advantages: ETM classes are fun and sociable. A well-designed class will provide you with comprehensive fitness training, and the observation of a good teacher ensures that you exercise safely and effectively. Adaptations and alternatives should be offered throughout the class to ensure all exercises are appropriate for your specific needs.

Disadvantages: It is vital that you check out the credentials of the teacher before attending an ETM class. A poorly constructed class, taught badly, can be unsafe and ineffective. Generally speaking, classes run by sports centres, fitness clubs and leisure centres only employ properly qualified teachers, but there is no guarantee. For advice on qualifications to look for, contact YMCA Fitness Industry Training (see Appendix 2). Your training is obviously restricted to the days and times that classes run. This limitation especially applies to those classes that only run during term time (common when run by adult education initiatives). Beware of becoming competitive with others when exercising with a large group of people in this way. Be sure to listen to your own body and exert yourself accordingly.

Unsuitable: Classes designed specifically for older adults, and run by qualified teachers, will be adapted to suit you whatever your special needs. The only conditions that are likely to make any ETM class a challenge are severe hearing or sight difficulties.

NB: Be sure to find a class to suit your level of fitness; this is important, as the degree of exertion required varies enormously. Classes are usually advertised as beginners, intermediate or advanced. If you are in any doubt, talk directly with the teacher of the class or, better still, attend the first one as an observer.

Opportunity: These classes are run at leisure centres throughout the country. Adult education initiatives also provide ETM classes. Individual teachers, using village halls, church halls and community centres, also run these classes independently. Your local library is likely to have all the contact details you will need. There are many ETM classes, specifically run for older adults, throughout the country.

Cost: Classes typically cost between £2.50 and £4.50. Some classes specifically for older adults can be even cheaper.

Free Weights

Description: The use of hand-held dumbbells and barbells (not machines) to develop muscular strength and endurance.

For Training Aerobic Fitness: Not effective, or appropriate. Due to the strain it places on your joints, and the likelihood of momentum throwing your body out of alignment, it is inappropriate to attempt to jog, run, dance or undertake any other form of dynamic aerobic exercise while holding free weights. The only exception to this is the use of light hand or wrist weights when walking, to train the endurance of your arm and shoulder muscles. Ankle weights may also be used for walking, providing that you are not overweight and do not have arthritis in your feet or ankles, or have bunions.

For Developing Muscular Strength: Potentially highly effective.

For Developing Muscular Endurance: A very effective way to train your muscular endurance.

For Increasing/Maintaining Flexibility: Not effective.

For Training of Motor Fitness: All strength training will develop your reaction time. A degree of coordination is required for some exercises, but correct technique is primarily dependent upon body awareness.

Equipment and Gear Needed: It is advisable to wear fitness shoes when using free weights, due to the risk of dropping one on your foot.

Advantages: Working with free weights is a far more natural way to develop your strength and endurance than sitting with your torso relaxed and supported by a machine while your arms and legs work. Using free weights with correct technique requires strength throughout your body, including your torso. This means that your core strength will increase as the strength of your limbs develops. This type of exercise can be easily tailored to target specific muscle groups according to your personal needs. Free weights are not expensive to buy, take up little storage space, and can be used within the comfort and convenience of your own home.

Disadvantages: It is vital that you learn, from a qualified fitness teacher, how to perform the exercises with correct technique, before attempting to do them alone at home. The incorrect use of free weights can result in serious injury.

Unsuitable: If you have significant arthritis in your hands, be sure to use weights with a wide grip. If the arthritis is severe then this type of exercise may be unsuitable for you. If you have high blood pressure or angina, or suffer from transient ischaemic attacks (ITAs), then avoid strength work altogether, and focus instead on developing muscular endurance. In the case of Parkinson's disease, strength training is best avoided. Light endurance work, accompanied by an extensive amount of stretching, is recommended instead. If you have severe kyphosis, a programme of exercises with free weights will need to be designed for you by a fitness teacher who is specifically qualified to work with such conditions.

Opportunity: You can use free weights in your own home and they are also provided by almost all fitness, sports and leisure centres and clubs.

Cost: The cost of a pair of dumbbells depends on their weight and the quality of manufacture. On average, prices range from £7–£20. Barbells are more expensive – the bars themselves range from £25–£75 and the discs to attach to them from £20–£50 for a set of four pairs.

Gardening

Description: Growing plants of any description, and/or landscaping. Whilst gardening is not an activity undertaken specifically for the exercise benefits it can bring, due to the diversity of movements potentially involved, it can provide a good all-round level of functional fitness.

For Training Aerobic Fitness: Typically, none of any significance.

For Developing Muscular Strength: This depends on the type of gardening you are doing. Heavy digging and moving rocks are examples of strength-demanding activities.

For Developing Muscular Endurance: With the exception of the lightest form of gardening, your endurance will be exercised to a greater or lesser degree.

For Increasing/Maintaining Flexibility: Bending down, reaching up and reaching out to the side are all movements that will help to maintain your ranges of functional movement. Unless you are reaching to the limit of a movement range for an extended duration, however, gardening will not actually increase your flexibility.

For Training of Motor Fitness: Some gardening activities require balance; in some instances a quick reaction time is necessary and occasionally coordination is challenged. These opportunities are, however, rare. Overall, gardening does not challenge your motor skills sufficiently to train them.

Equipment and Gear Needed: Obviously this varies enormously depending on what type of gardening you are doing. There are numerous books to help get you started.

Advantages: Gardening provides one of the most valuable forms of stress management known. It also, typically, involves being outside in the fresh air and natural light. Gardening is a highly creative pastime and can bring about rich rewards that far exceed fitness benefits alone. Similar to dance, the creative process of gardening can become the point of focus, rather than primarily a means to exercise.

Disadvantages: The degree of gardening activity you do may be strongly influenced by the weather and, therefore, may be only a seasonal form of exercise. Gardening is notorious for resulting in lower back pain. This is almost entirely avoidable if correct lifting and bending techniques are learnt from a qualified fitness teacher.

Unsuitable: Clearly, if you already have any sort of lower back pain, you will need to approach gardening with extreme caution and learn how to use your back without further damaging it. If you suffer from arthritis in your knees and/or hips, kneeling may be difficult and painful for you. If you have a hip replacement, seek advice from your physiotherapist or doctor regarding the appropriateness of kneeling or squatting. Modern-day hip replacements typically allow for far greater ranges of safe movement than those done years ago, but you still need specific clarification for your own personal case. Light gardening is good for arthritic hands as it helps to keep the joints mobile. If you have severe kyphosis, avoid crouching over low ground, as this will exacerbate the problem. Gardening in a greenhouse, conservatory or from raised beds, whereby you are gardening from an upright position, will suit you much better.

Opportunity: If you do not have your own garden, allotments are readily available to rent or buy in most locations. You do not even need to have your own garden in order to enjoy this wonderful pastime. Neighbours and friends often greatly appreciate help with their gardens. In addition, throughout the country there are conservation projects that rely on volunteer help for the preservation and maintenance of local areas of countryside. The exertion involved in such projects can be quite challenging, so it is best to ask beforehand what your participation would involve.

Cost: There is almost no limit to the amount of money that you could spend on your garden, if you chose to do so. In contrast, gardening can actually save you money if you grow your own food.

Golf

Description: A sport involving the propelling of a small hard ball with clubs across landscaped greens, in order to drop it into a series of small holes in the ground.

For Training Aerobic Fitness: If you walk rather than ride in a golf cart from one hole to the next, then golf can provide the opportunity for a walk. Unless your aerobic fitness is very poor, the intensity of the walking will not challenge your cardio-respiratory system.

For Developing Muscular Strength: Golf demands significant strength in the muscles of the shoulders, the chest, backs and fronts of the upper arms (one on one side, one on the other) and abdominals (external obliques).

For Developing Muscular Endurance: The only muscular endurance involved results from any walking you do, and is therefore limited to the lower body.

For Increasing/Maintaining Flexibility: Golf demands considerable flexibility of the shoulders and also the lower back (quadratus lumborum), abdominals (external obliques), and sides of upper back (latissimus dorsi).

For Training of Motor Fitness: A good degree of hand–eye coordination and special awareness is required to play golf.

Equipment and Gear Needed: Golf shoes, clubs, caddy and balls.

Advantages: Golf can offer social opportunities, is nonstrenuous and encourages time spent outside in fresh air and natural light. Due to the potential walking involved and the use of muscles in the upper torso, it is an excellent sport if you are recovering from heart disease.

Disadvantages: The specific muscles strengthened, and those made more flexible, by playing golf are not bi-lateral but one-sided, depending on whether you are right- or left-handed. Due to the twisting action involved in hitting a golf ball, the game places considerable strain on the lower back and knees.

Unsuitable: If you have severe arthritis in your feet, knees or hips, golf is inappropriate for you. If arthritic hands make holding the narrow grip of a golf club painful, consider widening the grip by covering it in many layers of tape, or purchasing a specially designed widening grip. If you suffer from osteoporosis or have lower back pain, golf is also contraindicated, because it places stress on your lumbar vertebrae. A frozen shoulder will prevent you from playing this sport. Due to the rotation of the hips that occurs with momentum when playing golf, it may not be a suitable activity if you have had a hip replacement. It is best to discuss your individual case with a physiotherapist. Although severe eyesight problems may render this sport impossible for you to play, many cases of moderately poor vision can be improved by repeatedly looking into the distance, as occurs when playing golf. Severe kyphosis can be exacerbated by the position needed for a golf swing. If you have bunions, the slight pivoting on the ball of the foot as you swing a club may be painful for you.

Opportunity: In the UK and most of Europe, golf courses exist within a reasonable driving distance of almost all geographical areas.

Cost: Golf equipment is relatively expensive to buy but can usually be hired from clubs. Inexpensive second-hand clubs can sometimes be found at charity shops or advertised for sale in your local newspaper. Memberships to golf clubs vary but are typically more expensive than many other sports clubs.

Jogging/Running

Description: Jogging is a term typically used to describe a gentle run with minimal elevation off the ground. It is performed at a consistently steady pace. Running is a fast dynamic pace involving long strides and significant impact as the feet hit the ground.

For Training Aerobic Fitness: Both jogging and running are superb cardio-respiratory conditioners.

For Developing Muscular Strength: The only strength work involved is in the legs if running up very steep hills.

For Developing Muscular Endurance: An excellent way to develop endurance in the muscles of your legs and hips.

For Increasing/Maintaining Flexibility: Ineffective – in fact, muscles in the legs and hips tend to shorten if this activity is not balanced with plenty of stretching.

For Training of Motor Fitness: Speed can be trained if sprinting is included. If you are running off-road on uneven terrain, then balance and reaction time will also be challenged.

Equipment and Gear Needed: A good pair of running shoes is essential. Clothing needs to be non-restrictive, breathable and layered.

Advantages: Both running and jogging are movements that are totally natural to the human body. These activities can be done in almost any geographical location at zero cost, other than the investment in proper shoes. The impact involved helps to maintain the integrity of the pelvic floor, strong bones and healthy lymphatic functioning. Jogging and running provide an excellent opportunity to be outside in the fresh air and natural sunlight. Becoming adept at running enhances your personal safety.

Disadvantages: Due to the impact involved, these activities are unsuitable for a number of conditions (see below). In some geographical locations personal safety may be a concern. Fair weather exercisers may find that wet conditions frequently interrupt their training programme. All non-yielding man-made surfaces, such as concrete and tarmac, are unnatural. If you ran on such surfaces with bare feet, this would result in excessive trauma to your bones and joints. By wearing well-designed running shoes, you can largely reduce the impact of road running, but extensive amounts of road running is still unhealthful. The more you can run off-road the better.

Unsuitable: Jogging and running are unsuitable if you have significant arthritis in any of your weight-bearing joints (feet, ankles, knees, hips or lower back). Although these activities are an excellent way to keep bones strong, if you already have osteoporosis the impact can further damage your bones and even cause fractures. Having a weak pelvic floor does not mean that you cannot take up jogging. It simply means that you need to build up to it gradually by mixing walking with a few paces of jogging to begin with. Jogging and running are both unsuitable if you suffer from significant lower back pain or have had a hip replacement. If you are significantly overweight, you need to lose the weight before taking up these activities, as the impact will be too great for your joints to withstand. If you have severe kyphosis, power walking (see page 239) will be better for you than jogging or running, as your spine will have reduced shock absorbency. Do not jog or run if you have a detached or partially detached retina. Jogging and running are also unsuitable if you currently have a whiplash injury. The presence of bunions will probably make either activity painful for you. If you attempt to run with bunions, the adapted posture you might adopt may be detrimental to your lower knees, hips and lower back.

Opportunity: Almost anywhere you go you will find somewhere you can run or jog. Even most cities have a number of parks. There are running clubs in most areas and, if you are concerned about personal safety, running with others is an answer.

Cost: The only costs involved are running shoes, appropriate clothing and, if you choose to join a running club, your subscription.

Pilates

<u>Description</u>: Pilates comprises of very specific exercises designed to strengthen the muscles of your torso (primarily your abdominals and your back), thus creating superior stability of your core (pelvis and spine). Pilates can be done with machines or on a mat on the floor. It is the floorwork version that we will be looking at here.

<u>For Training Aerobic Fitness</u>: None.

<u>For Developing Muscular Strength</u>: Very effective at developing stronger abdominals and pelvic floor muscles.

<u>For Developing Muscular Endurance</u>: Develops endurance throughout the body.

<u>For Increasing/Maintaining Flexibility</u>: Ranges of movement are comprehensively maintained by Pilates and some ranges can be developed. Improvements in posture and mechanical use of the body contribute significantly to greater freedom of movement throughout the body.

<u>For Training of Motor Fitness</u>: Body awareness is the key to Pilates. Coordination is also required.

<u>Equipment and Gear Needed</u>: Non-restrictive clothing that allows your bodyline to be seen by your teacher. An exercise mat.

<u>Advantages</u>: Developing powerful core stability needs to be the first step for anyone interested in improving their fitness. No matter what other sports or activities you plan to undertake, the practising of Pilates will render your performance more effective and safer. Pilates can reduce back pain, or even bring about total relief.

<u>Disadvantages</u>: None, other than the need to undertake some additional form of exercise in order to train your cardio-respiratory system.

<u>Unsuitable</u>: If you have high blood pressure, then be sure to seek the guidance of a qualified Pilates teacher and inform them of your condition, as there are some movements that will be inappropriate for you. If you have had a hip replacement you can still practise Pilates, but you will need to adapt it considerably. Be sure to seek advice about this. Due to the fact that much of the Pilates floorwork involves lying on your back, it will be inappropriate for you if you have severe kyphosis. An experienced and knowledgeable teacher will be able to offer you alternative positions.

Opportunity: Pilates has gained greatly in popularity during the last decade. Classes are run at many leisure, sports and recreation centres. Independent teachers also work from village halls and community centres. Your local adult education initiative will almost certainly run courses in Pilates. In some locations Pilates studios exist. Many books and videos are available, but it is recommended that you attend classes run by a qualified Pilates teacher before going it alone at home.

Cost: Classes can be expensive, depending upon where they are run.

Rebounding and Trampolining

Description: A trampoline consists of a bed suspended within a frame by springs. A full-sized trampoline is 7 feet by 14 feet and stands about 4 feet off the ground. Numerous smaller sizes are available for beginners and children. A rebounder is a mini trampoline that is small enough to fit in any average living space and light enough to stow away easily after use. Rebounders stand only a few inches high, but the elastic bed provides you with the opportunity to bounce your way into quite a sweat!

For Training Aerobic Fitness: Bouncing provides excellent aerobic exercise.

For Developing Muscular Strength: Overall, much depends upon the type of movements that are executed. Advanced trampolining demands a high degree of strength in a wide range of muscles and can include those of the upper body. Generally, however, the strength challenge when bouncing is predominantly to the lower body. At the level of a total beginner, there is virtually no challenge to actual strength at all.

For Developing Muscular Endurance: An excellent way to develop endurance in your legs and torso.

For Increasing/Maintaining Flexibility: Advanced trampolining demands considerable flexibility but does not develop it. An additional programme of developmental stretching is necessary if high levels of skill are to be achieved on the trampoline. Rebounding does not provide opportunities for greater flexibility.

For Training of Motor Fitness: There are few activities that train balance, coordination, reaction time and body and spatial awareness more effectively than trampolining and rebounding.

Equipment and Gear Needed: You do not need to have your own trampoline or rebounder to enjoy this activity. Coaching in trampolining is available at most sports and leisure centres, many of which run classes in rebounding. Investing in your own rebounder at home ensures availability of daily practice. Other than a very well-supporting bra for larger breasted women, there are no specific clothing requirements. Bare feet are the preferred choice for trampolining and rebounding. If you do have a very weak pelvic floor, your may need to wear a pad to catch any urine that escapes as you bounce.

Advantages: This is an excellent form of aerobic exercise for people with compromised bones or joints, as the landing surface is always highly yielding. Even if a significant degree of arthritis or osteoporosis is present, rebounding can still be appropriate. It stimulates the bone-building cells and promotes the production of joint fluids, without exerting excess force on vulnerable bone and joint structures. One of the greatest benefits of rebounding is the positive influence it exerts upon your lymphatic system. Your lymphatic fluids rely largely on changes in pressure in order to flow through your body. The G-force that results from bouncing creates such pressure changes and consequently is a powerful lymphatic booster. As your lymphatic system is responsible for your ongoing detoxification processes, this is a massive asset to the health of your entire body. In the absence of other influences, the less toxic you are, the less acid is your blood. Because the cause of osteoporosis is an overly acid bloodstream, having an efficient lymphatic system to help keep your blood pure can therefore be considered vital to strong and healthy bones. Bouncing on a rebounder is probably the most effective way to improve the tone and efficiency of your pelvic floor muscles. Due to the G-force of each landing, your pelvic floor has to contract or else urine may be passed. If this proves a problem, simply begin by bouncing very gently and then gradually progress the height of your bounce over the weeks as your pelvic floor strengthens.

This form of exercise is an excellent way to develop muscular endurance in your legs, as well as condition your heart, lungs and blood vessels, and improve your balance. Rebounding can be done in the comfort and privacy of your own home, in a small space, and with minimal set-up time. Many people enjoy bouncing to music. This is helpful as it encourages a rhythmical perfor-mance. Children find rebounding a whole lot of fun, so if you want a form of exercise you can enjoy with them, this is certainly one option. All in all, rebounding gets a very high rating!

Disadvantages: There are very few disadvantages to rebound-ing, other than it possibly becoming addictive because it is so much fun! There are dangers involved, especially with trampolin-ing, related to falling between the bed and the frame, or landing awkwardly. For this reason, even if you intend to invest in a trampoline at home it is best to obtain some coaching in basic safety and correct technique before you practise alone.

Unsuitable: If you have arthritis in your neck, bouncing is unsuitable for you. Bouncing is also contraindicated if you have vertigo or other balance problems, a detached or partially detached retina, current whiplash injury or are in moderate to advanced stages of Parkinson's disease.

If you suffer from lower back pain, bouncing might help your condition or worsen it, depending on the nature of your injury. Advice from a chiropractor will help you to identify your needs. Due to the risk of landing awkwardly, and the spontaneous wide steps that sometimes need to be taken in any direction, tram-polining is totally unsuitable if you have had a hip replacement. Gentle bouncing on a rebounder, placed in the corner of a room so that you have the walls either side of you to catch your balance is acceptable.

Opportunity: Most rebounders are made with legs that unscrew, meaning that should you spend time away from home you can take it in the car with you. If you would like to try one out before getting one of your own, then your local leisure centre probably has one that you can sample.

Cost: Trampoline classes typically cost £3.50–£5 per group session. Private coaching can be very expensive and may be over £50 per hour. Your local sports or leisure centre will be able to advise you as to the cost of private lessons. To purchase a tram-poline of your own will cost between about £350 and £12,000, depending on the size and the quality. The cost of rebounders varies considerably according to quality, and size, of the product. Prices range from around £40 to about £200. A rebounder in the

£60–£70 range will meet the needs of most home bouncers for many years.

Resistance Bands and Tubes

<u>Description</u>: Resistance bands are lengths of rubberized material, typically about 4–6 in (10–15 cm) wide and 4–6 feet (1–2 m) in length. They are available in various densities providing a range of resistances. Resistance tubes are lengths of tubular rubber, typically with a D-shaped handle at either end. Tubes are also available in a range of resistances.

<u>For Training Aerobic Fitness</u>: Not relevant.

<u>For Developing Muscular Strength</u>: Both bands and tubes can be used to train strength.

<u>For Developing Muscular Endurance</u>: Excellent endurance training equipment.

<u>For Increasing/Maintaining Flexibility</u>: Bands or tubes can be used to assist you in some stretch positions.

<u>For Training of Motor Fitness</u>: Not relevant (except if you have a great imagination and creativity).

<u>Equipment and Gear Needed</u>: As different muscles in your body have different degrees of strength and endurance, a set of three different resistances will be the most helpful to you.

<u>Advantages</u>: Bands and tubes take up very little space, are light to transport and ideal to take with you when travelling or away form home. They provide opportunities for a wide range of strength and endurance training and cost very little.

<u>Disadvantages</u>: If used incorrectly, or with poor technique, using these items can result in injury.

<u>Unsuitable</u>: If your hands are arthritic, the narrow grip required to hold the bands will render them unsuitable for you. To overcome this problem with tubes, padding may be wrapped around the handles to widen the grip. If you have high blood pressure, it is recommended that you avoid strength work and focus on developing your endurance instead. Some of the exercises will be inappropriate if you have a frozen shoulder. If you have lower back problems, be especially careful to practise correct technique. If you have severe kyphosis, seek the advice of a qualified fitness professional to show you exercises that will help to improve, rather than exacerbate, your condition.

Opportunity: Resistance bands and tubes are available at most sports shops (see also Appendix 2). Classes using bands and tubes are run at many sports and leisure centres.

Cost: Resistance bands are around £3.50–£5 each. Resistance tubes are around £5–£7 each.

Resistance Machines

Description: Machines individually designed to provide resistance to specific muscles, the degree of resistance being adaptable according to a person's needs. Multi-gyms consist of one unit that provides a range of exercises. There is typically some adjusting of pulleys/hooks/benches, etc. involved to change the exercise.

For Training Aerobic Fitness: None.

For Developing Muscular Strength: Very effective.

For Developing Muscular Endurance: Very effective.

For Increasing/Maintaining Flexibility: None.

For Training of Motor Fitness: None.

Equipment and Gear Needed: A pair of training shoes (cross-trainers are fine), and non-restrictive clothing that is reasonably close fitting, so as to run no risk of it getting caught in the machinery.

Advantages: Specific muscle groups can be isolated and targeted. Many machines provide an opportunity for overcoming high resistances without weight bearing on the feet, ankles, knees or hips.

Disadvantages: Resistance machines typically provide support for your torso while you exercise your arms and legs. A consequence of their frequent use is that you develop a weak torso and limbs that are stronger than your torso can stabilize. Resistance machines are expensive to buy and take up a large amount of space, so are generally not suitable for home use. Your exercise sessions are therefore governed by the opening hours of the venue where they are located. Resistance gyms are popular and therefore typically used by large numbers of people. This may result in you having to wait a significant time to use the machine of your choice. The complex technology of some machines may feel intimidating to you, as might the other users who may include some serious body builders. Whatever your physical condition, it is vital that you obtain clear instructions from a qualified fitness professional regarding the safe use of each machine before you attempt to use them unaided.

Unsuitable: If you have high blood pressure, avoid strength work and focus on developing your endurance. Some machines will be unsuitable for you if you have severe kyphosis.

Opportunity: Resistance gyms are found within most sports, recreation and leisure centres, as well as private gyms.

Cost: Some gyms require membership, which can vary from reasonable to expensive. Some local centres offer pay-as-you-go facilities, but will require you to undertake an initial induction to show you how to use the equipment. If not, initially you will need to invest in the services of a qualified fitness professional to show you how to use the machines safely. If you have the space, and choose to create your own gym at home, a simple multi-gym can be as cheap as £300–£500. There is virtually no upward limit on the amount you can spend.

Squash

Description: A racket sport played indoors by two or four people, in a wall-enclosed court. Squash involves hitting a small rubberized ball against a wall.

For Training Aerobic Fitness: The bouts of exertion in squash are intense and short-lived, thus making it an anaerobic sport and not effective for training aerobic fitness.

For Developing Muscular Strength: Strength in the arm and shoulder of the playing arm is required. Leg strength is also developed to a lesser degree, depending on your skill level.

For Developing Muscular Endurance: As bouts of exertion are typically only for short durations, squash is not effective for training endurance.

For Increasing/Maintaining Flexibility: Flexibility of the playing shoulder and hips is needed to play squash, but the game itself will not develop flexibility. It is advisable to develop your flexibility via regular yoga practice, to minimize your risk of injury when playing.

For Training of Motor Fitness: A super way to develop quick reactions.

Equipment and Gear Needed: Squash shoes, a squash racket

and balls. Balls are available for different speeds of play. If you are a beginner, be sure to start with the slowest balls.

Advantages: Due to the speed and intensity of exertion, squash can be a good outlet for acute stress. It is the one racket sport that, even if you cannot find a partner to play with, you can go into a court and practise alone. The development of anaerobic fitness does have advantages, enhanced personal safety being one of them.

Disadvantages: Due to the speed and intensity of squash, it is common for people to sustain injuries such as pulled muscles. To minimize the risk of this, it is advisable to develop a good all-round level of fitness before taking up this sport. It is also common for squash to be the preferred sport of chronically stressed-out business people. Because such people typically have high blood pressure, this is a poor match, as squash will elevate blood pressure further during play. Upper body strength is only developed on the side of the playing arm. The overall fitness benefits of squash are limited.

Unsuitable: Squash is unsuitable if you have any of the following conditions: significant arthritis anywhere in your body, high blood pressure, a frozen shoulder on your playing arm, lower back pain, hip replacement(s), knee replacement(s), obesity, fibromyalgia, Parkinson's disease, a detached or partially detached retina or a current whiplash injury. Depending on your style of play, bunions may or may not make squash an uncomfortable activity for you.

Opportunity: Most sports, leisure and recreation centres have squash courts for hire. Squash clubs also exist throughout the country.

Cost: To hire a court at a public sports facility typically costs between £3.50–£5.50 per hour.

Step Classes

Description: Stepping repeatedly on and off a low platform, using a variety of foot patterns and some arm movements, accompanied by music.

For Training Aerobic Fitness: Provides powerful aerobic training. This form of exercise also demands moderate to high levels of reaction time and coordination.

<u>For Developing Muscular Strength</u>: Exercises to train strength are not typically included in a step class.

<u>For Developing Muscular Endurance</u>: Step develops substantial endurance of your leg muscles and, depending on the choreography, can challenge the endurance of your arms too.

<u>For Increasing/Maintaining Flexibility</u>: A well-designed step class will include a comprehensive range of maintenance stretches towards the end of the class. Developmental stretches are not typically incorporated.

<u>For Training of Motor Fitness</u>: Step significantly challenges co-ordination and requires some degree of balance. If you are following a teacher's choreography, your reaction times will also be tested.

<u>Equipment and Gear Needed</u>: You will need a pair of exercise shoes and loose fitting, breathable and comfortable clothing. Dress in layers so that you can remove items of clothing as you get hot. Be sure to take water with you to drink; this type of exercise can cause you to sweat a considerable amount.

<u>Advantages</u>: Step is very effective at challenging your cardio-respiratory system due to the extensive use of the large muscles of your thighs and hips. It can also be fun as it is performed to music and is an effective way to develop your coordination.

<u>Disadvantages</u>: It is not at all mechanically natural for your body to repeatedly step up onto, and then down from, a step. Stepping is renowned for leading to repetitive stress injuries of the knees and lower back. For this reason, if you choose to include this type of exercise in your regimen, you are strongly advised to not participate in stepping more than once a week. Unless you have a good degree of coordination, you are at risk of falling over your own feet, or tripping over the step.

<u>Unsuitable</u>: If you have significant arthritis in your knees, hips, or lower back, stepping is contraindicated. If you suffer from vertigo or other balance problems, step is also unsuitable. Definitely avoid stepping if you have any type of lower back or knee pain.

<u>Opportunity</u>: Step classes are typically run at most leisure centres.

<u>Cost</u>: Attending a step class will probably cost you £3–£5.

Swimming

<u>Description</u>: Using the body to move through water without touching the ground.

<u>For Training Aerobic Fitness</u>: An excellent cardiovascular conditioner.

<u>For Developing Muscular Strength</u>: Some strokes, such as butterfly, challenge strength when sprinted over a short distance.

<u>For Developing Muscular Endurance</u>: A superb whole-body endurance challenge.

<u>For Increasing/Maintaining Flexibility</u>: A good degree of flexibility, especially of the shoulders, is required to swim well. Swimming itself, however, does not develop flexibility.

<u>For Training of Motor Fitness</u>: Coordination is key in swimming.

<u>Equipment and Gear Needed</u>: None except a swimsuit, a towel and possibly a pair of goggles. Some public swimming facilities require you to wear a swimming cap. Additional equipment such as floats for added resistance when performing strength and endurance work, are an optional extra. These may be provided by some public pools or you might prefer to purchase your own.

<u>Advantages</u>: Swimming is, mechanically, a totally natural pastime for your body. It can provide an excellent aerobic training solution if you suffer from any type of joint pain, or are considerably overweight. This is because it does not involve any weight bearing on your joints. Swimming does involve the exertion of a comprehensive range of your muscles, and it is something that you can enjoy with your children and grandchildren, without anyone needing to wait for another to catch up, as may be the case with walking or cycling.

<u>Disadvantages</u>: If you live in a location where the ocean is clean and warm enough to swim in, then you are most fortunate. The alternative use of public swimming baths certainly has the major disadvantage of exposing your body to highly toxic chemicals put in the water in an attempt to control micro-organisms. Swimming also typically involves travelling to the water, which may be a disadvantage if transport is a problem. Of course, if you have the luxury of your own swimming pool at home, both of these disadvantages are negated!

<u>Unsuitable</u>: Many swimming strokes will be a problem if you suffer from severe arthritis in your neck or have a current whiplash injury. A frozen shoulder, or a significant open wound, will temporarily render swimming unsuitable. If you are epileptic, be sure never to swim alone.

<u>Opportunity</u>: This very much depends upon your location unless, of course, you are fortunate enough to have your own pool. Most towns and villages are less than ten miles from a public swimming facility.

<u>Cost</u>: The use of public swimming facilities is typically not expensive. Some leisure facilities offer subsidized swimming for older age groups.

Tai Chi

<u>Description</u>: A form of martial arts, involving sequences of very slow, flowing and controlled movements.

<u>For Training Aerobic Fitness</u>: None.

<u>For Developing Muscular Strength</u>: None.

<u>For Developing Muscular Endurance</u>: Effective for developing the ability to sustain slow and controlled movements.

<u>For Increasing/Maintaining Flexibility</u>: Tai Chi involves a variety of movement ranges, some of which are take the joints to their full range. It is an effective way to maintain flexibility but will not develop it.

<u>For Training of Motor Fitness</u>: A very effective way to develop balance, coordination and body awareness.

<u>Equipment and Gear Needed</u>: None other than non-restrictive clothing.

<u>Advantages</u>: Due to the very slow speed of the movements, tai chi encourages physical confidence. This can result in people achieving greater movement ranges than they would attempt at a faster pace. This is especially true for people with significant joint pain, such as arthritics and people with Parkinson's disease. Tai chi is also an excellent form of movement if you suffer from stress.

<u>Disadvantages</u>: There are no disadvantages to tai chi other than the fact that you would need to undertake other activities in order to train your cardiovascular fitness and strength. If you need to develop your flexibility, then you will also need to spend time separately working on that.

Unsuitable: If you have severe arthritis of the knees, you might find that tai chi does not suit you. Although there is no deep knee bending involved, a significant bend in the knees is used for most movements.

Opportunity: Once experienced, you can practise tai chi on your own anywhere. Initially, however, it will serve you best to attend classes to learn the sequences and correct technique. Some sports, leisure and recreation centres run classes. Sessions are also available at martial arts centres and courses are commonly run by adult education initiatives. Your local library can probably advise you about classes available in your area.

Cost: Classes typically cost between £2.50 and £4.50.

Tennis

Description: A racket sport played on a court with a central net, by two or four players.

For Training Aerobic Fitness: If the goal is to keep a rally going, then tennis can be an effective way to maintain your aerobic fitness, but this will not be possible until you have reached a moderate level of skill. For beginners, tennis is a very stop-start activity with insufficient sustained movement to challenge your aerobic system. Tennis matches, played by experienced players, consist of some short bouts of activity and some extended periods of play. Overall, tennis can be considered an aerobic/anaerobic activity depending on the skill level of the players and the way the game develops.

For Developing Muscular Strength: Strength is required in the muscles of the playing arm and shoulder. The more skilled a player you become the more strength is required, and the more muscles become involved. Leg strength is also developed in dynamic play, and especially in singles matches as you have to lunge to reach balls at the limits of your range.

For Developing Muscular Endurance: Rallying is a good way to develop endurance in your leg muscles.

For Increasing/Maintaining Flexibility: The more skilled you become at tennis, the greater is your need to be flexible. The game itself will not develop your flexibility, so it is advisable also to practise yoga to minimize your risk of injury when playing.

For Training of Motor Fitness: Excellent for training eye-to-ball coordination, reaction time, coordination, speed and agility.

Equipment and Gear Needed: Tennis shoes, a racket, tennis balls and non-restrictive clothing. Some clubs have a strict dress code and may only allow the wearing of white clothing.

Advantages: Tennis is fun, sociable and has a wide range of fitness benefits. Playing on the non-yielding surface of a hard court is useful for keeping your bones strong.

Disadvantages: The necessity of a partner may sometimes prevent you from playing, although if you join a club that problem is usually easily overcome. In some facilities it is possible to hire a tennis wall, which is designed for solo practice. Although indoor courts are available, tennis is typically played outside, rendering it a fair weather activity.

Upper body strength is developed on the side of your playing arm only. Additional exercise needs to be done on your non-playing arm to achieve physical balance. Excessive play can result in an overuse injury to the elbow of your playing arm.

Unsuitable: If you have severe arthritis in your feet, knees, hips, playing hand or neck, tennis may be unsuitable for you. Playing on a grass court may alleviate the problem to some degree. If you have a frozen shoulder on your playing arm, you cannot play tennis, unless you choose to develop ambidextrous skills. Bunions on your feet may make tennis uncomfortable for you.

Opportunity: Many sports, leisure, and recreation centres have tennis courts for hire. Tennis clubs exist throughout the country.

Cost: The hire of a court at a public facility typically costs between £3 and £5 per hour. Club memberships can be expensive, but it varies from area to area.

Walking and Hiking

Description: Walking that is continually sustained for an extended period, relative to a person's fitness. Hiking is usually done off-road and often incorporates an undulating landscape.

For Training Aerobic Fitness: Trains your aerobic fitness, providing that your walking pace and the terrain that you cover are appropriate for challenging your level of fitness.

For Developing Muscular Strength: None, except if you are walking up exceptionally steep inclines.

For Developing Muscular Endurance: An excellent endurance trainer for the muscles of your legs. There is no significant muscular challenge from the pelvis up.

For Increasing/Maintaining Flexibility: None as such, but due to a tendency for the muscles at the front of your hip (hip flexors) to lose flexibility as you get older, your stride length will gradually shorten. Counteract this by aiming to walk with a longer stride.

For Training of Motor Fitness: There is a minimal coordination and balance requirement that would not be sufficient to challenge you unless you are severely debilitated.

Equipment and Gear Needed: Although you can have fun kitting yourself out with a variety of clothing designed for the purpose, a comfortable pair of walking shoes and a good pair of socks is all that is essentially required. Depending on your familiarity with your intended route, a map and/or a compass may be necessary. Waterproof clothing is a good idea to take with you in inclement weather.

Advantages: Walking can be done at any time of day and in almost any location. It is the most natural mechanical action for your body. You can easily vary the intensity from moment to moment, according to how you are feeling. Walking costs nothing other than the investment in a good pair of walking shoes. It provides an opportunity for you to access fresh air and sunshine, and can be a very social activity if you walk with others. It can also provide you with some time for constructive thinking and therefore help you to better manage stress. Walking can be of additional practical use, such as walking to perform an errand, and therefore can reduce petrol costs and environmental damage through car emissions. Walking, and especially hiking, provide an excellent degree of skeletal trauma to help your bones stay strong, and it is therefore highly recommended if you have concerns about osteoporosis. If you have severe osteoporosis, then avoid uneven ground.

Disadvantages: There are few disadvantages to walking, with the possible exception of your personal safety if you do it alone in certain areas. It is important to gradually progress the intensity or duration of your walking over the weeks, otherwise your fitness will only develop so far and then level off. If walking with others, ensure that you choose people whose fitness level is similar to yours.

Unsuitable: If you have significant arthritis in your feet, knees or hips, shorter and more frequent walks are recommended. Lower back pain should not be exacerbated by walking, provided that you maintain good posture as you do so.

Opportunity: Everywhere you go there are opportunities to walk.

Cost: No cost unless you take public transport to your starting point.

Yoga

Description: Depending on the type of yoga, how you approach it, who your teacher is, and what your personal needs are, yoga can be an entire philosophy of living and deeply spiritual way of life, or it can be reduced to nothing more than a series of stretches.

For Training Aerobic Fitness: With the exception of advanced performance of dynamic types of yoga (such as Ashtanga), the aerobic challenge of yoga is virtually nil.

For Developing Muscular Strength: Strength is needed in order to achieve some of the more advanced postures.

For Developing Muscular Endurance: For most forms of yoga, endurance is required to hold postures for an extended period of time. However, this requires low-grade static endurance (isometric), as opposed to the ability of your muscles to repeatedly bring about dynamic movements (isotonic), as is practically useful in everyday life. The type of endurance involved in yoga can, though, result in significant improvements in your posture.

For Increasing/Maintaining Flexibility: The regular practising of yoga is one of the very best ways to increase your flexibility.

For Training of Motor Fitness: Few other activities can develop your balance as effectively as yoga.

Equipment and Gear Needed: Non-restrictive clothing that allows your bodyline to be seen by the teacher. Possibly a yoga mat, although most classes held at leisure and sports centres provide these.

Advantages: Yoga is a superb way to learn to manage your stress better. It can help you if you suffer from insomnia and can be adapted to suit anyone, regardless of how debilitated or out of condition they may be. Regular yoga practice can improve your posture, and dramatically improve your flexibility. It is highly recommended for everyone.

<u>Disadvantages</u>: There are very few disadvantages to yoga other than the fact that in order to maintain or develop your cardio-respiratory fitness, you would need to partake in an additional form of exercise.

<u>Unsuitable</u>: Yoga can be adapted to be suitable for all special needs. Seek the advice of a qualified yoga teacher if you have any specific conditions.

<u>Opportunity</u>: Yoga classes are run by almost all sports, leisure and recreation centres. Independent teachers in village and community halls also run many classes. There are plenty of excellent books and videos to assist you in practising yoga, but you really need to work with a teacher to begin with until you have mastered performing the basic postures with the correct technique.

<u>Cost</u>: Classes vary in price, but typically cost between £3 and £5.

Appendix 1
Commonly Used Drugs and their Implications for Exercise

Because the body of an older person is, on average, significantly lower in water than that of a youngster, any given dose of medication will be more concentrated within their system and will also take longer to clear from their bloodstream. An appropriately modified dose, according to age, is more important when using some drugs than others. The typically slower processing of drugs needs to be taken into consideration if medication and exercise are being programmed in relationship to each other.

Analgesics (Painkillers)
Used for: Pain relief. (In the case of non-opioid analgesics, for pain relief and/or to reduce a fever. In the case of non-steroid anti-inflammatory drugs, for pain relief and/or to reduce a fever and/or to reduce inflammation.)

General Implications for Exercise
Pain is one of your body's ways of communicating its needs to you. If pain is felt, it is likely to be a sign that some degree of rest and immobility is needed. In cases where a problem has become chronic it may sometimes support healing to move, regardless of the pain. If analgesics are being taken to reduce inflammation, it may or may not be appropriate for you to exercise at all. It is vital that you seek the advice of your doctor or health care provider on the above issue. Never exercise if you have a fever.

The most common side-effects of analgesics are constipation, nausea, vomiting, dizziness, indigestion, drowsiness and headaches. Long-term use of these drugs typically results in some degree of fluid retention, which manifests as swollen ankles and feet. If you experience breathing difficulties or black or blood-stained bowel movements at any time while taking analgesics, discontinue them immediately and seek medical advice.

- All analgesics reduce your body awareness and your ability accurately to perceive how hard you are exerting yourself during exercise. They will also interfere with your ability to identify the onset of any exercise-induced pain and compromise your awareness of the limitations of your joint and muscle ranges. If you are taking painkillers, keep your exercise within moderate limits of intensity
- Exercise is one of the most effective ways to solve problems with constipation
- Dizziness will reduce your proprioception (the unconscious perception of movement and spatial orientation arising from stimuli within the body itself) and your ability to balance
- If drowsy, you may lack the desire to exercise and/or tire quickly when you do
- If you are on stronger analgesics such as morphine and consequently experience confusion, do not attempt to undertake any type of activity that requires concentration or complex techniques
- Exercising out of doors in the fresh air may help to alleviate headaches
- Be especially careful to avoid exercising after a meal to minimize indigestion
- Exercise may help alleviate the fluid retention that can result from taking these drugs.

Antacids

Used for: Indigestion, heartburn, inflammation or ulceration of any of the upper portions of the intestinal tract or stomach.

General Implications for Exercise

- *Aluminium compounds* interfere with phosphate absorption. This leads to muscle weakness and contributes to causing osteoporosis. These effects need to be taken into consideration when planning any progressive fitness programme. If you habitually take these drugs, you need to minimize all other potential causes for osteoporosis and regularly participate in activities that are bone strengthening (see Chapter Seven). Aluminium compounds may also cause constipation. Regular exercise can be a great help in alleviating this

- *Magnesium compounds* are likely to cause muscular weakness. They also stress the kidneys, so it is especially important to keep well hydrated when being physically active. These drugs also cause drowsiness and lethargy, making exercise more of an effort and premature fatigue likely
- *Sodium Bicarbonate* These drugs result in excess sodium circulating in the blood, which is likely to cause a rise in blood pressure. If you are taking these drugs, avoid activities that dramatically increase your blood pressure further, such as isometrics, strength work and explosive activities. The increase in sodium will also cause water retention (oedema). Regular aerobic exercise can help to alleviate this. These drugs also predispose you to bloating, which can make abdominal exercises or lying on your stomach uncomfortable to perform and inhibit your breathing.

Anti-angina Drugs
Used for: Angina.

General Implications for Exercise
This category of drugs includes beta-blockers (see page 249), calcium channel blockers, nitrates and potassium channel openers. Due to causing dilation of the blood vessels, as a general rule all anti-angina drugs are likely to result in dizziness, especially when moving from a lying-to-sitting or sitting-to-standing position. For this reason care should be taken during any activities where such changes in body positioning are being made, as fainting is possible. The dilation of the blood vessels also results in a flushed appearance to the skin. This renders evaluating the intensity of your exertion according to your complexion less accurate. Swelling of the ankles may occur when taking these drugs. Keeping the ankles regularly mobile through movement can help to alleviate this. If you have been prescribed anti-angina drugs,

you should heed the exercise advice offered in Chapter Seven, under Exercise for Cardiovascular Health.

Anti-arrhythmics

Used for: Arrhythmia (erratic/irregular heartbeat).

General Implications for Exercise

These drugs affect the normal functioning of the heart. As a consequence, dizziness when moving from lying-to-sitting or sitting-to-standing and/or breathlessness when physically active may result. Headaches and nausea are also possible outcomes of taking anti-arrhythmics, which may make exercising unappealing.

The drug amiodarone accumulates in the tissues of the body and can lead to lung problems and light-sensitive rashes. Care should therefore be taken when participating in outdoor activities under strong sunlight and medical advice should be sought if any difficulties with breathing occur. Gains or losses in body weight may be attributable to changes in thyroid function because of using this drug. If attempts are being made to lose or gain weight through diet and/or exercise, this needs to be taken into consideration.

Antibiotics

Used for: Infections.

General Implications for Exercise

In the case of antibiotics, it is not so much the drug but the reason you are taking it that needs to be considered. Antibiotics are prescribed to combat infections. Depending on the site and type of infection you have, it may be unwise for you to exercise at all until it is resolved. Seek your doctor's advice on this.

Swimming in a public pool is contraindicated with any external infection, as are activities where there is potential body contact with another person at the point of infection. Significantly raising your body temperature through vigorous activity can be counter-productive to healing infections. Exercise creates a significant increase in your blood circulation, which can result in infections spreading more rapidly. Whenever your body is working to overcome an acute crisis such as an infection, it is rest, not activity, which is needed.

Anticoagulants

Used for: Reduction in aspects of the blood's clotting factors to reduce the likelihood of blood clots forming.

General Implications for Exercise

Warfarin and heparin are the most commonly used oral anticoagulants. The primary potential side-effects involve haemorrhaging and all such signs should be reported to your doctor immediately. Contact sports are contraindicated for anyone taking these drugs, due to the possibility of internal bleeding or clot formation. If you have been prescribed an anticoagulant you should take the exercise advice offered in Chapter Seven, under Exercise for Cardiovascular Health.

Anti-diabetic Drugs

Used for: Diabetes.

General Implications for Exercise

The three primary groups of anti-diabetic drugs are:

- *Sulphonylurea* Encourages the pancreas to produce insulin
- *Metformin* Alters the way sugar is metabolized by the body
- *Acarbose* Slows the digestion of starches.

Ascertaining the correct dose for any of these drugs is not easy. Too much sulphonylurea can result in an excessive lowering of blood sugar, resulting in hypoglycaemia. Due to the influence of a typically varied diet, what is the appropriate amount of medication one day may prove to be too much the next. During exercise the body's use of blood sugar increases and decreases parallel to the intensity of the physical exertion. It is therefore necessary to monitor the situation closely, by maintaining a high level of body awareness whenever being significantly physically active. Sulphonylurea can also negatively affect the blood cell count. If this occurs, it will have a significant detrimental influence on your energy levels and aerobic capacity.

There is no danger of hypoglycaemia when using metformin, but it commonly causes nausea, weight loss, abdominal distension and diarrhoea. It is therefore difficult to ascertain if any alterations in total body weight that occur are due to exercise, diet or the influence of the drug.

If acarbose is used and the dose is not altered in accordance with patterns in fitness training, there is a possibility that insufficient fuel will be available when needed for the more intense phases of exercise.

Antihypertensive Drugs
Used for: Hypertension (high blood pressure).

General Implications for Exercise
The six primary groups of antihypertensive drugs are:

- *Centrally acting drugs* Affect the brain and consequently its dictations for vascular dilation
- *Beta blockers (see page 249)* Render the heartbeat weaker
- *Diuretics (see page 251)* Reduce blood volume by interfering with the function of the kidneys
- *ACE inhibitors* Affect enzymes in the blood that influence the dilation of blood vessels
- *Vasodilators (see page 255) and calcium channel blockers* Inhibit the contraction of the walls of the arteries
- *Alpha blockers* Block the transmission of messages for blood vessels to constrict.

For specific implications of beta-blockers, diuretics and vaso-dilators, please refer to the individual entries on the following pages. The general side-effects of all antihypertensive drugs are that of dizziness and fainting due to the reduction in blood pressure. Care should therefore be taken when moving from a standing-to-sitting or sitting-to-standing position. The primary consideration is that if you have been prescribed any of these drugs, you need to address the cause (see Chapters One and Two) and take the exercise advice offered in Chapter Seven under Exercise for Cardiovascular Health.

Anti-rheumatic Drugs

Used for: Various rheumatic disorders including rheumatoid arthritis and gout.

General Implications for Exercise

- Taking any anti-rheumatic drugs places your kidneys under stress, so it is especially important to keep well hydrated
- High or prolonged doses of chloroquine can cause eye damage. Get your eyes checked regularly, especially if you participate in sports where your safety is dependent upon your vision
- If you are taking immunosuppressants, seek the advice of your doctor before undertaking any type of regular vigorous physical activity
- If you are taking gold-based drugs, they can suppress the production of blood cells from your bone marrow. This has implications for your aerobic potential.

Beta-blockers

Used for: Angina, hypertension, irregular heartbeat, migraines, anxiety, hyperthyroidism.

General Implications for Exercise

These drugs have a powerful impact upon many systems of the body, including:

- *Heart* Weakens and slows the contractions of the heart muscle
- *Respiratory tract* Constricts the airways
- *Blood vessels* Causes them to constrict including those that surround the brain.
- *Blood pressure* Is lowered.

As beta-blockers have such a powerful effect on the heart, circulation and breathing, their use renders many standard approaches to monitoring fitness training invalid. In addition, constriction of the blood vessels and respiratory passageways inhibits the passage of oxygen and blood to the skeletal muscles. This results in a reduced anaerobic threshold, while simultaneously compromising the body's ability to process lactates produced by anaerobic performance. The overall effect is one of severely compromised fitness potential.

If you have been prescribed beta-blockers for angina or hypertension, you need to address the causes of your condition (see Chapters One and Two) and take the exercise advice offered in Chapter Seven, under Exercise for Cardiovascular Health. If taking these drugs for anxiety, remember that regular vigorous exercise is an effective and healthful approach to coping with such a problem.

Bronchodilators

Used for: Asthma and bronchitis.

General Implications for Exercise

There are three main groups of these drugs: sympathomimetics, xanthine and anticholinergics.

- *Sympathomimetics* and *xanthine* can affect the heart rate, sometimes causing palpitations. This needs to be considered when monitoring your heart rate during exercise, and it can be misleading if you are evaluating your fitness progress by charting your resting heart rate
- *Anticholinergics* can cause eyesight problems, so it is advisable to have your vision checked regularly. This is important if you participate in activities whereby your safety is especially dependent upon clear vision.

Corticosteroids

Used for: All types of arthritis, strains, sprains, frozen shoulder, bursitis, tendonitis and contracted muscles.

General Implications for Exercise

The potential side-effects of corticosteroids are many and their use can be severely detrimental to your health. When used as a one-off treatment it is likely that you are looking for a quick fix. You would be far better off to take the necessary time to rest and allow your body to heal itself naturally.

If you are considering long-term use of these drugs, then you should weigh up the benefits and the risks with your doctor in accordance with your own specific case. Long-term use of corti-costeroids will result in a gradual deterioration in your capacity to exercise as your overall health declines.

Digitalis
Used for: Irregular heartbeat, atrial fibrillation, congestive heart failure, post heart attack.

General Implications for Exercise
This drug reduces the efficiency of the nervous impulses within the heart muscle that dictate its speed of contraction. It also causes the heart to contract more forcefully with each beat. As digitalis alters the functioning of your heart, the use of it invalidates many standard approaches to monitoring aerobic fitness training, such as heart rate monitoring. The toxic qualities of digitalis become more dangerous to the body when potassium is low. For this reason it is vital when participating in activities that require a high intensity of exertion, or take place in hot environments, that you replace lost potassium. Eating bananas is the simplest and most effective way to achieve this. If you have been prescribed digitalis, you need to address the causes of your problem (see Chapters One and Two) and follow the exercise advice offered in Chapter Seven under Exercise for Cardiovascular Health.

Diuretics
Used for: Oedema (water retention), hypertension (high blood pressure), heart failure, nephritic syndrome (a kidney disorder), cirrhosis of the liver, premenstrual syndrome, glaucoma, Meniere's disease.

General Implications for Exercise

- The most common problem with diuretics is hypokalaemia (loss of potassium). For this reason it is vital when participating in activities that require a high intensity of exertion, or take place in hot environments, that you replace lost potassium. Eating bananas is the simplest and most effective way to achieve this
- Many types of diuretics cause an accumulation of uric acid within the body. This may manifest as gout. Uric acid

accumulation can also cause muscular pain and soreness that is unrelated to physical exertion

- Blood sugar levels may rise under the influence of diuretics. Exercise can help to normalize blood sugar and prevent drug-induced hyperglycaemia
- When using diuretics there is an increased risk of becoming dehydrated during physical exertion, especially in hot or humid environments. If you use these drugs, ensure that you keep well hydrated
- Diuretics typically cause a feeling of general malaise, which may reduce your desire to exercise
- If you are using diuretics for high blood pressure, then you need to address the causes of your problem (see Chapters One and Two) and take the exercise advice offered in Chapter Seven under Exercise for Cardiovascular Health.

Gallstone Drugs

Used for: Gallstones.

General Implications for Exercise

The two main drugs used are chenodeoxycholic acid and ursodeoxycholic acid. The most common side-effect is diarrhoea. As these drugs need to be taken over an extended duration in order to bring about changes in gallstones, the greatest potential risk is chronic dehydration as a result of chronic diarrhoea. Keeping fluid intake high, especially when exercising, therefore becomes vitally important. These drugs also result in elevated cholesterol levels in the blood. Because of this particular side-effect, blood pressure should be monitored and exercise adapted accordingly (see Chapter Seven under Exercise for Cardiovascular Health). Luckily these days ultrasound and surgical techniques are available as two alternatives for dealing with gallstones, so drugs are rarely used.

Glaucoma Drugs

Used for: Glaucoma.

General Implications for Exercise

Drugs used include miotics, beta-blockers (see page 249) and diuretics (see page 250). If you are using miotic eye drops, you may find it challenging to see in poor light. If this is the case, avoid activities that take place indoors in poorly lit environments or out of doors after sunset or before sunrise. The use of any diuretics will result in a more frequent need to urinate and increased thirst, which needs to be borne in mind before you undertake certain long distance/long duration activities. A feeling of general malaise is also common when taking diuretics, which can reduce your desire to be physically active.

Lipid-lowering Drugs

Used for: Hyperlipidaemia (excess fats in the blood), diabetes, post heart attacks.

General Implications for Exercise

If you have been prescribed these drugs for hyperlipidaemia or because you have had a heart attack, you need to address the cause (see Chapters One and Two) and then take the exercise advice offered in Chapter Seven under Exercise for Cardiovascular Health. One common side-effect of lipid-lowering drugs is constipation. Exercise can help to alleviate this. Many types of these drugs also cause a reduced ability for the body to absorb fat-soluble vitamins. As vitamins A and E are a vital part of your defences against damage from free radicals, it is especially important to avoid exercising in polluted atmospheres such as cycling in heavy city traffic. Lipid-lowering drugs stress both your kidneys and your liver to some degree. Because of this, ensure that you keep well hydrated when exercising.

Muscle Relaxant Drugs

Used for: Muscular contractions that can occur with osteoarthritis, back problems or injury; or muscular spasticity resulting from conditions such as multiple sclerosis, stroke or cerebral palsy.

General Implications for Exercise

- Drowsiness can result in poor technical performance, which has implications for injury risk. If you are taking these drugs, avoid activities that are high-risk, such as contact sports, and those whereby your safety depends upon complex/specific technique such as using free weights

- If using these drugs, your muscles will to some degree be compromised in their ability to contract and allowances for your performance need to be made accordingly.

Osteoporosis Drugs

Used for: Osteoporosis (some of the same drugs are used for osteomalacia, rickets and Paget's disease).

General Implications for Exercise

Numerous drug approaches are taken to treating osteoporosis including: Calcitonin (a hormone), hormones taken from enforcedly impregnated female horses (called Premarin), mineral and vitamin preparations (calcium and vitamin D) and bisphosponates (such as etidronate – Didronel – and alendronate).

None of these drugs have direct implications for exercise, but most have side-effects that may render exercising more challenging.

- *Etidronate* Can cause diarrhoea, nausea, constipation, abdominal pain, rash and itching
- *Premarin* Can cause vomiting, weight loss or gain, swelling and tenderness of the breasts and oedema (fluid retention).

Parkinsonism Drugs

Used for: Parkinson's disease.

General Implications for Exercise

These drugs are designed to restore the balance between two organic compounds in the body – dopamine and acetylcholine. They are divided into two categories: those that reduce the effects of acetylcholine (anticholinergics) and those that increase the effects of dopamine (dopamine-boosting drugs).

There are no specific implications with regard to exercising while using these drugs. The side-effects, however, need to be taken into account, as they can render exercising more challenging.

- *Anticholinergics* Can cause dry mouth, blurred vision, difficulty in passing urine, agitation, constipation, dizziness, confusion, nausea, vomiting, nervousness, rash*, itching*, palpitations*
- *Dopamine-boosting drugs* Can cause loss of appetite and nausea. Other possible side-effects include headaches*, muscular pain*, dizziness*, rash*. If you are experiencing Parkinson's disease, you are best to seek the guidance of a qualified fitness teacher who can design an appropriate exercise programme for you according to you own specific needs and abilities.

NB: *If you experience these side-effects, see your doctor immediately.

Vasodilators
Used for: Hypertension (high blood pressure), atherosclerosis, arteriosclerosis, angina, peripheral vascular disease, senile dementia.

General Implications for Exercise
These drugs relax the muscles of the blood vessels, causing the vessels to widen. The most common side-effect is that of dizziness and fainting due to a significant drop in blood pressure. Care should therefore be taken when changing body positions from lying-to-sitting or sitting-to standing and activities that repeatedly require such postural changes, such as judo, should be avoided. Flushing is also very common and so evaluating physical exertion according to the complexion becomes invalid. These drugs can also cause oedema (fluid retention). Exercise can help to alleviate this to some degree. Vasodilators typically predispose the user to headaches, which increased physical exertion can sometimes make worse.

For more on any of the drugs listed above, and for details of drugs not mentioned, see *The British Medical Association's Concise Guide to Medicines and Drugs*. ISBN 0-7513-0466-2.

Appendix 2
Useful Resources

Equipment

Nottingham Rehab Ltd.
Ways & Means
Sindel House
Excelsior Road
Ashby Park
Ashby De La Zouch
Leicestershire LE65 1NG
Tel: 0845 606 0911
Website: www.nrf-uk.co.uk

Suppliers of a wide variety
of equipment to assist in
rehabilitation and for use by
people with special needs.
Products include those
useful for daily living for
people with compromised
mobility.

Physical Company
2a Desborough Industrial
Park
Desborough Park Road
High Wycombe
Buckinghamshire HP12 3BG
Tel: 01494 769 222
Email:
sales@physicalcompany.co.uk
Website:
www.physicalcompany.co.uk

Suppliers of all manner of
fitness equipment for home or
commercial use. Excellent
mail order service.

ProActive Health Limited
Quarry Court
Bell Lane
Cassington
Oxon OX29 4DS
Tel: 0870 8484 842
Email:
info@proactive-health.co.uk
Website:
www.proactive-health.co.uk

Suppliers of a very wide
range of fitness equipment,
monitors and educational
material. Mail order
service.

General Support for Older Adults

Age Concern
Astral House
1268 London Road
London SW16 4ER
Tel: 020 8765 7200
Helpline: 0800 009966

Website:
www.ageconcern. org.uk

Provides a wide range of
support and resources for
older adults and works closely
with national, regional and
local organiZations. Age
Concern also initiates many
national projects, including
Ageing Well UK.

Health and Fitness

Aquarobics

YMCA Fitness Industry Training
111 Great Russell Street
London WC1B 3NP
Tel: 0207 343 1850

Fitness Professionals
University of East London
Longbridge Road
Dagenham
Essex RM8 2AS
Tel: 0870 5133434
Useful website:
www.aquafunfitness.com/
aquarobicslinks.html

Badminton

Badminton Association of England Ltd.
National Badminton Centre
Bradwell Road

Loughton Lodge
Milton Keynes MK8 9LA
Tel: 01908 268400
Website: www.baofe.co.uk

Bowls

English Bowling Association
Lyndhurst Road
Worthing
West Sussex BN11 2AZ
Tel: 01903 820222
Website:
www.bowlsengland.com

Callisthenics

Keep Fit Association
Astra House
Suite 105 Arklow Road
London SE14 6EB
Tel: 020 8692 9566
Website: www.keepfit.prg.uk

YMCA Fitness Industry Training
111 Great Russell Street
London WC1B 3NP
Tel: 020 7343 185

Fitness Professionals
University of East London
Longbridge Road
Dagenham
Essex RM8 2AS
Tel: 0870 5133434
Website for products
www. callisthenics.co.uk

Circuit Training

Fitness Professionals
University of East London
Longbridge Road
Dagenham
Essex RM8 2AS
Tel: 0870 5133434
Useful website: www.circuit
trainingdirectory.com

YMCA Fitness Industry Training
111 Great Russell Street
London WC1B 3NP
Tel: 020 7343 185

CR/CV Gym

Fitness Professionals
University of East London
Longbridge Road
Dagenham
Essex RM8 2AS
Tel: 0870 5133434

Gym World
Head Office
120/122 Yorkshire Street
Oldham
Lancashire
OL1 1ST
Tel: 0800 018 5294
Website:
www.gymworld.co.uk

YMCA Fitness Industry Training
111 Great Russell Street
London WC1B 3NP
Tel: 0207 343 1850

For products

Simply Fitness Kybotech Ltd.
The Garden Room
Church Lane
Carlton-on Trent
Newark
Nottinghamshire NG23 6LP
Tel: 0870 777 8891
Website: www.simplyfitness
equipment.co.uk/Gym
Equipment

Cricket

England and Wales Cricket Board
Lord's Cricket Ground
London NW8 8QZ
Tel: 020 7432 1200
Website: www.ecb.co.uk

Cycling

British Cycling Federation
National Cycling Centre
Stuart Street
Manchester M11 4DQ
Tel: 0870 871 2000
Website:
www.britishcycling.org.uk

Dancing

The British Association of Teaching Dancing
23 Marywood Square
Glasgow
Scotland G41 2BP
Tel: 0141 423 4029
Website: www.batd.co.uk

British Dance Council
(Ballroom dancing)
Terpsichore House
240 Merton Road
South Wimbledon
London SW19 1EQ
Tel: 020 8545 0085
Website:
www.british-dance-council.org

English Folk Dance
Cecil Sharp House
2 Regent's Park Road
London NW1 7AY
Tel: 020 7485 2206
Website: www.efdss.org

Imperial Society of Teachers of Dancing
Imperial House
22-26 Paul Street
London EC2A 4QE
Tel: 020 7377 1577

International Dance Teachers' Association
International House
76 Bennett Road
Brighton BN2 5JL
Tel: 01273 685 652

The Laban Guild for Movement and Dance
22 Welbeck Avenue, High Brooms
Tunbridge Wells
Kent TN4 9BD
Tel: 01892 537 077

Margaret Morris Movement
The International Association of MMM Ltd.
PO Box 1525
Helensburgh
Dunbartonshire G84 0AF
Tel: 01934 420 241
Website: www.margaret morrismovement.com

Medau Movement
8b Robson House
East Street
Epsom
Surrey KT17 1HH
Tel: 01372 729056
Website: www.medau.org.uk

Royal Academy of Dance
36 Battersea Square
London SW11 3RA
Tel: 020 7326 8000
Website: www.rad.org.uk

Exercise to Music

Extend
2 Place Farm
Wheathampstead
Hertfordshire AL4 8SB
Tel: 01582 832760
Website: www.extend.org.uk

Fitness Professionals
University of East London
Longbridge Road
Dagenham
Essex RM8 2AS
Tel: 0870 5133434

Keep Fit Association
Astra House
Suite 105
Arklow Road
London SE14 6EB
Tel: 020 8692 9566
Website: www.keepfit.prg.uk

YMCA Fitness Industry Training
111 Great Russell Street
London WC1B 3NP
Tel: 0207 343 1850

Free Weights

Fitness Professionals
University of East London
Longbridge Road
Dagenham
Essex RM8 2AS
Tel: 0870 5133434

YMCA Fitness Industry Training
111 Great Russell Street
London WC1B 3NP
Tel: 020 7343 185

Gardening

The Royal Horticultural Society
Pershore Group of Colleges
Avonbrook
Pershore
Worcestershire WR10 3JP
Tel: 01386 552 443
Website: www. Pershore.ac.uk

Golf

Ladies Golf Union
The Scores
St Andrews
Fife KY16 9AT
Tel: 01334 475811
Website: www.lgu.org
Useful website:
www. golfcourses.org

The Royal and Ancient Golf Club of St Andrews
Golf Place
St Andrews
Fife
KY16 9JD
Tel: 01334 60000
Website: www.randa.org

Jogging/running

UK Sport
40 Bernard Street
London WC1N 1ST
Tel: 020 7211 5100
Website: www.uksport.gov.uk
Useful websites:
www. runnersworld.co.uk
www.runnersweb.co.uk/
indexrun.htm

Pilates

**The Body Control Pilates
Association**
6 Langley Street
Covent Garden
London WC2H 9JA
Tel: 020 7379 3734
Website:
www.bodycontrol.co.uk

Rebounding/Trampolining

Dr Douglas Graham
1 Cassidy Place
Storrington
West Sussex RH20 4EY
Tel: 01903 746572
Website:
www. foodnsport.com
Useful website:
www. trampoline.co.uk

Resistance Bands and Tubes

Fitness Professionals
University of East London
Longbridge Road
Dagenham
Essex RM8 2AS
Tel: 0870 5133434
Website for products
www.callisthenics.co.uk/

Keep Fit Association
Astra House
Suite 105 Arklow Road
London SE14 6EB
Tel: 020 8692 9566
Website: www.keepfit.prg.uk

**YMCA Fitness Industry
Training**
111 Great Russell Street
London WC1B 3NP
Tel: 020 7343 185

Resistance Machines

Fitness Professionals
University of East London
Longbridge Road
Dagenham
Essex RM8 2AS
Tel: 0870 5133434

Gym World
Head Office
120/122 Yorkshire Street
Oldham

Lancashire OL1 1ST
Tel: 0800 018 5294
Website: www.gymworld.co.uk

YMCA Fitness Industry Training
111 Great Russell Street
London WC1B 3NP
Tel: 020 7343 185

For products

Simply Fitness
Kybotech Ltd.
The Garden Room
Church Lane
Carlton-on Trent
Newark
Nottinghamshire NG23 6LP
Tel: 0870 777 8891
Website:
www. simplyfitnessequipment.
co.uk/GymEquipment

Squash

England Squash
National Squash Centre
Rowsley Street
Manchester M11 3FF
Tel: 0161 4384317
Website:
www.englandsquash. com

Step Classes

Fitness League
6 Station Parade
Sunningdale
Berkshire SL5 0DP
Tel: 01344 874787
Website:
www.thefitnessleague.com

Fitness Professionals
University of East London
Longbridge Road
Dagenham
Essex RM8 2AS
Tel: 0870 5133434

YMCA Fitness Industry Training
111 Great Russell Street
London WC1B 3NP
Tel: 020 7343 185

Swimming

Amateur Swimming Association
Harold Fern House
Derby Square
Loughborough
Leicestershire LE11 5AL
Tel: 01509 618700
Website:
www.britishswimming. org

Tai Chi

Martial Arts Development Commission
PO Box 461
Wembley
Middlesex HA0 3WD
Tel: 0870 7700461

Tai Chi Union
1 Littlemill Drive
Balmoral Gardens
Crookston Glasgow
G53 7GF
Tel: 0141 810 3482
Website: www.taichiunion.com

Tennis

Lawn Tennis Association
Palliser Road
London W14 9EG
Tel: 020 7381 7000

Walking and Hiking

The Rambler's Association
2nd floor Camelford House
87-90 Albert Embankment
London SC1 7TW
Tel: 020 7339 8500
Website: www.ramblers.org.uk

Yoga

The British Wheel of Yoga
25 Jermyn Street
Sleaford
Lincolnshire NG34 7RU
Tel: 01529 306851

The Sivananda Yoga Vedanta Centre
51 Felsham Road
London SW15 1AZ
Tel: 020 8780 0160

Professor Rozalind Graham

Health Consultant
Email: rozgruben@aol.com/
healthyunlimited@aol.com
Website:
www.rawmatriark.com

Professor Graham (author of this book) is available for personal consultations regarding health, nutrition, fitness, lifestyle, and emotional health, and speaking appointments.

Dr Douglas Graham

Website:
www.foodnsport.com
Dr Graham provides personal training, education, fitness programmes and lifestyle coaching for athletes and health seekers of all ages.

The Central Council of Physical Recreation (CCPR)

This is an excellent overall resource. It is an umbrella for the national sporting and recreation governing bodies, representing and promoting their interests. If you cannot access the information you need about any specific sport or activity, the CCPR will be able to help you. When it comes to the cost of various activities, remember that if you are a senior citizen most sports and leisure centres will offer you a considerable discount.
Contact details: Francis House, Francis Street, London SW10 1DE.
Tel: 0207 8548521.
Website: www.ccpr.org.uk

Healthful Living International (HLI)
PO Box 595
Sebastopol CA 95473
USA
Website:
www.healthfulliving.org

HLI is a non-profit organization promoting healthful living throughout the world. HLI provides education, resource information, and support, as well as seminars and a regular newsletter, in order to teach people how to heal themselves through healthful living.

Nutrition and Diet

EarthSave International
PO Box 96
New York NY 10108
USA
Tel: (001) 718 459 7503
Website: www.earthsave.org

Promotes a plant-based diet for superior health, environmental support and animal rights. EarthSave provides education materials and seminars and also runs hundreds of local groups around the world.

European Vegetarian Union (EVU)
E-mail: evu@ivu.org
Website: www.ivu.org/evu

Promotes vegetarianism throughout Europe, providing information, contacts and resources. The EVU also runs congresses.

The Fresh Network
PO Box 71
Ely
Cambridge CB6 3ZQ

Tel: 0870 800 7070
E-mail:
info@freshnetwork.com
Website:
www.fresh-network. com

Promotes the raw diet by providing information, support and running events. The Fresh Network also runs a substantial mail order service selling various products.

International Vegetarian Union (IVU)

Tina Fox
c/o The Vegetarian Society
UK
Parkdale
Durham Road
Altrincham
Cheshire WA14 4QG
Tel: 0161 925 2002
Website: www.ivu.org

The IVU has an extensive website providing a wide range of information on vegetarianism, upcoming events, recipes, and other organizations. The IVU works to promote vegetarianism throughout the world.

The Vegan Society

Donald Watson House
7 Battle Road
St. Leonards on Sea
East Sussex TN37 7AA
Tel: 01424 427393
Website:
www.vegansociety.com

The Vegan Society promotes veganism and provides education, information, contact details of other organizations, recipes, books, and many other services. Their mission is to teach people how to live free from animal products for the benefit of health, animals and the environment.

The Vegetarian Society of the United Kingdom

Parkdale
Dunham Road
Altrincham
Cheshire WA14 4QG
Tel: 0161 925 2000
Website: www.vegsoc.org

Providing comprehensive education, support and resources for all those interested in leading a vegetarian lifestyle.

Organics

Henry Doubleday Research Association

Ryton-on Dunsmore
Coventry CV8 3LG

Tel: 024 7630 3517
Website: www.hdra.org.uk

Promotes all aspects of organic gardening. Publishes practical information. Provides products and runs a seed bank.

Soil Association
Bristol House
40-56 Victoria Street
Bristol BS1 6BY
Tel: 0117 929 0661
Website:
www.soilassociation.org

Promotes and conducts research in organic farming and gardening. Publishes the *Soil Association Quarterly Review*.

Special Needs

British Blind Sport
4-6 Victoria Terrace
Leamington Spa
Warwickshire CV31 3AB
Tel: 01926 424247
Website:
www.britishblindsport. org.uk

Provides information and support for anyone with impaired vision who would like to take part in sport or leisure activities of any sort.

British Wheelchair Sports Foundation
Guttmann Road
Stoke Mandeville
Bucks HP21 9PP
Tel: 01296 395995
Website: www.bwsf.org.uk

This organization provides information and support for wheelchair athletes and wheelchair users who want to partake in sports and recreational activities.

UK Sports Association for People with Learning Disability
Leroy House
436 Essex Road
London N1 3QP
Tel: 0870 770 2464
Website:
www. uksportsassociation.org

Provides information and support for anyone who has a disability and wants to participate in sport of any sort.

References and Bibliography

Chapter 1: Creating a Healthy Lifestyle
1 A.C. Neilson Company; Louis Harris Poll 1993.
2 Belin LJ. Vegetarian diet and blood pressure levels: incidental or casual association. Am J Clin Nutr 1988;48:806–10.
3 Rouse IL, Armstrong BK, Belin LJ, Vegetarian diet, lifestyle and blood pressure in two religious populations. Clin Exp Pharmacol and Physiol 1982;9:327–30.

Mind Body Medicine, Daniel Goleman, PhD and Joel Gurin, Consumer Reports, 1993

Love, Medicine and Miracles, Bernie Siegel M.D., Arrow, 1986.

Life 101, John-Roger and Peter Mc Williams, Thorsons, 1992.

Quantum Healing, Deepak Chopra, M.D., Bantam,1989.

Why People Don't Heal, Caroline Myss, Boulder, 1994.

Basic Clinical Science, Dr Nic Rowley, Hodder and Stoughton, 1991.

Smoking The Facts, Health Education Authority, 1991.

Passive Smoking at Work, Health and Safety Executive, IND(G) 63(L) revised C1000 1/93.

Reversing Heart Disease, Dr Dean Ornish, Ballantine Books.

Health Update 2 – Smoking, Health Education Authority, 1991.

Please Don't Smoke in Our House, Jack Dunn Trop, NH Press, 1976.

A Consumers Guide to Stop Smoking, Penny Ross PhD/Sarah Hack BSc., 1990.

The Smoking Epidemic, The Health Education Authority, 1993.

Living Health, Diamond, Bantam Books, 1987.

The China Study: The Most Comprehensive Study of Nutrition Ever Conducted and the Startling Implications for Diet, Weight Loss and Long-Term Health, T. Colin Campbell, Thomas M. Campbell II, Benbella Books, 2005.

Food For Life: How the New Four Food Groups Can Save Your Life, Dr. Neal Barnard, Three Rivers Press, 1994.

The Food Revolution: How Your Diet Can Help Save Your Life and Our World, John Robbins, Conari Press, 2001.

McDougall's Medicine: A Challenging Second Opinion, Dr. John A. McDougall, New Win Publishing, 1986.

Chapter 2: A Time for Change
Physical Dimensions of Ageing, Waneen W. Spirduso, Human Kinetics.
Exercise Programming for Older Adults, Kay A Van Norman, Human Kinetics.
London Central YMCA Training and Development Department Teacher Training Manual. The British Medical Association, Dorling Kindersley.

Chapter 5: Ready, Steady, Go!
Physical Dimensions of Ageing, Waneen W. Spirduso, Human Kinetics.
Exercise Programming for Older Adults, Kay A Van Norman, Human Kinetics.
London Central YMCA Training and Development Department.
'Osteoporosis', Susie Dinan and Dr Olga Rutherford PhD. MSc. BA. ASSET March 1994.
The British Medical Association, Dorling Kindersley.

Chapter 7: Choosing Your Fun and Where to Find It
Dr Nicholas A DiNubile, The Physician and Sports Medicine, July 1997, Vol 25, No.7, pp 47–56.
Johns & Wright, 1962.
Ekdahl & Broman, 1992.
Liang, 1992.

Index

diabetes (*cont.*)
  diet and 15
  obesity and 17, 186
  risk factors 17, 57
  type 2 diabetes 15
diet 15–19, 265–6
  calorie requirement 18, 188
  comfort eating 195–6
  disease and 15, 179–80, 183
  excess fat 16–17
  food addiction 195
  fruit and vegetables 16, 17, 195
  healthy diet 15–16, 187–8
  organic food 16, 267
  overeating 5, 7, 16, 18–19, 195–6
  salt 16
  toxins 35
  vegetarian 2, 15, 265–6
  weight-loss diets 187
  whole foods 15–16, 188
digestive problems
  obesity and 17
  posture and 45
digestive system 5, 13, 16
  exercising and 85
digitalis 251
disabilities, people with 267
diuretics 248, 251–2, 253
Dorsal Raises 110–12, *111, 112*
driving 3, 7
dumbbells 71, 72, 98, 221

elbow joints 88
embolism 181
emotional health 7, 8, 9–10
  emotional upsets 95
  heart health and 9
  negative emotional states 9, 56
emphysema 12, 31
endocrine system 32–3
  see also hormonal activity

endurance training 27, 28, 41–2, 57
  duration 82–3
  exercises 114–68
  fat burning 57, 191
  frequency 82
  intensity 82
  see also individual activities
energy 61–2, 196
eosinophilia 9
epinephrine 8
equipment 86–7, 98, 194, 257
exercise
  instructions 96–168
  and longevity xi
  and medication 243–55
  national fitness survey (1992) 37
  and specific health conditions 169–202
  sports and recreational activities 203–42
  see also fitness training
exercise area 86
eyesight impairment 30–1, 46

falls 43, 58, 86, 198
fat, body 17–18, 33, 42, 57
  fat burning 57, 188–95
fat, dietary 16–17, 35
fatigue 19
fibre 16
Fight or Flight Response 8, 62
fitness
  cardio-respiratory fitness 38–40
  evaluating 63–6
  flexibility 42
  law of specificity 70, 77
  motor fitness 43
  muscular endurance 41–2
  muscular strength 40–1

Daily Telegraph Health series

Encyclopedia of Vitamins, Minerals & Herbal Supplements

Dr Sarah Brewer
1-84119-184-1
£9.99

The most comprehensive and up-to-date review of vitamins, minerals, herbal remedies and other nutritional supplements.

A bewildering range of vitamin, mineral and herbal supplements is now widely available to us all, but information about their health benefits cannot be given on the packaging as it would constitute a health claim. In this jargon-free guide, leading expert on sensible supplementation, Dr Sarah Brewer, sets out all you need to know about the main supplements, and suggests what to take for specific health problems.

- A–Z guide to 150 supplements for a brighter and healthier life
- Clearly explains the benefits, possible side-effects and contraindications
- Thoroughly sets out the research evidence to back their efficacy
- Recommends supplements for common problems such as IBS, chronic fatigue, recurrent candida and arthritis

Packed with clear and concise answers, this essential guide explains the use of supplements to maintain or improve your daily health.

See order form on the back page to order a copy now and save £2!

Daily Telegraph Health series

The Family Encyclopedia of Medicine & Health

1-84119-898-6
£12.99

Answer all your questions about health in a way you really understand with this fully updated edition, which has new sections on weight control, polycystic ovarian syndrome, fibromyalgia and fatigue.

- Huge range of entries, covering both common and unusual medical terms and problems
- Includes entries for major symptoms and treatments
- Full and up-to-date descriptions for each entry
- Cross-referenced to direct you to related entries or give further information
- Helpful illustrations showing parts of the body and how most of the major organs work
- Jargon-free, clearly arranged and easy to read

'Useful in several different ways – in providing simple explanations for technical terms, in offering a guide to the cause and treatment of common conditions and especially in supplying the sort of background information that will allow you to understand medical matters that affect you and your family.' Dr James Le Fanu, *The Daily Telegraph*

'The definitive medical reference book.' *My Weekly*

'An ideal reference for the home.' *Your Health Care Magazine*

See order form on the back page to order a copy now and save £2!

Daily Telegraph Health series

Arthritis
The complete guide to relief using methods that really work

Arthur C. Klein
1-84529-073-9
£9.99

New updated and revised edition of the arthritis bestseller.

Those who have arthritis know there is a world of difference
between the treatments that doctors recommend and the
treatments that actually work in practice. This bestselling book is
based on public surveys in which arthritis sufferers were asked
what best relieved their symptoms and improved their quality of
life. Surgery? Nutrition? Exercise? Alternative therapies? You'll
find the answer to this and many more questions in this book.

In this revised and updated text incorporating the results from a
2005 UK survey, you will find:

- Conventional treatments, surgery and drugs
- Experimental treatments
- Pain-relieving techniques
- Alternative therapies
- Self-help techniques, organizing your life and home
- Nutritional advice, including diet and 30-day meal plan
- Exercise: nearly 200 pages of illustrated and effective exercise
  plans

'Here, uniquely, those with arthritis can learn from the
experiences of others. That is what makes this a truly
excellent book.' Dr James Le Fanu, *The Daily Telegraph*

**See order form on the back page to order a copy now and
save £2!**

Order further Daily Telegraph health titles and save £2 on every title

Title	RRP	Offer price	Qnty	Total
Alzheimer's Disease	£7.99	£5.99		
Crohn's Disease & Ulcerative Colitis	£9.99	£7.99		
Epilepsy	£9.99	£7.99		
Food Medicine	£9.99	£7.99		
Sleep Really Well	£9.99	£7.99		
Arthritis	£9.99	£7.99		
Encyclopedia of Vitamins, Minerals & Herbal Supplements	£9.99	£7.99		
Home Doctor	£9.99	£7.99		
Family Encyclopedia of Medicine & Health	£12.99	£10.99		
Depression	£9.99	£7.99		
Hip Replacement	£9.99	£7.99		
Complete Guide to Allergies	£9.99	£7.99		
P&P				£1.00
Grand Total				£

Name: _____

Address: _____

_____ Postcode: _____

Daytime Tel. No. / Email _____

Three ways to pay:

1. **For express service telephone the TBS order line on 01206 255 800 and quote 'BPHD'. Order lines are open Monday – Friday 8:30am – 5:30pm**
2. I enclose a cheque made payable to **TBS** Ltd for £
3. Please charge my □ Visa □ Mastercard □ Amex □ Switch (switch issue no. .....)
   £ _____
   Card number:
   Expiry date: _____ Signature _____
   (your signature is essential when paying by credit card)

Please return forms (no stamp required) to, Constable & Robinson Ltd, FREEPOST RLUL-SJGC-SGKJ, Cash Sales/Direct Mail Dept, The Book Service, Colchester Road, Frating, Colchester CO7 7DW. All books subject to availability.

Enquiries to: readers@constablerobinson.com
www.constablerobinson.com

Constable & Robinson Ltd (directly or via its agents) may mail or phone you about promotions or products. Tick box if you do not want these from us □ or our subsidiaries □